The

1ˢᵗ Aisle

How to Eat for
MAXIMUM HEALTH

Kirk Charles

Library of Congress Cataloging-in-Publication Data
ISBN: **0-9836080-1-6**
ISBN-13: **978-0-9836080-1-1**
Printed in the United States of America

Contents

Table of Contents

Note to the Reader

Once at the gym a friend walked by and said, "Hey Kirk, long time no see. Whatcha been up to?" I replied, "Just tryin' to stay young!" We smiled at each other and kept moving.

Over the last 30 years, staying young is all I've been working on. I have not quite figured it out yet, but many of my clients have told me I have been able to slow down the aging process just a tad. For me, staying young is about athleticism, accomplishment and attitude. Those qualities are generally viewed as being in the domain of the youthful, and often associated with increased energy. Yet, I attempt to instill them in my clients through targeted exercise and results oriented eating, regardless of age. At its core, staying young is about the efficiency of your metabolism, not whether it is fast or slow. When your metabolism is firing on all cylinders, it can release you from the throes of disease and provide a much smoother journey through life. This is accomplished simply by giving your body what it needs for fuel and breaking a sweat at the gym, outside or in the comfort of your home.

The 1st Aisle is an easy, step-by-step process that keeps you younger and more vibrant through the power of whole food plant-based eating. As you read further you may not agree with all that is expressed on the topics of health and eating, but a little dissent here and there keeps things interesting. Some of my clients and critics have called me controversial, crazy, sadistic, overzealous, unrealistic and flat out wrong—while some have even said I am quite charming. How I love them all! Their reactions deepen my knowledge, expand my experience, and reinforce my core philosophy: *those who eat predominantly from the first aisle get superior results.* I have seen it time and time again. Without doubt, fresh produce from the first aisle is the alpha and omega of energy and vitality.

Meet you in the first aisle,

Kirk

Preface

Running with my good buddies Ilya, Brad, Andrea, Wezi and Patrick is always a highlight for me—they are better conditioned than I am, and they push me to the limit. My goal is to just keep up; and oftentimes I'm barely hanging in there. Many times I've wanted to sit down, give up and cry, but they would not stand for that. Even when I am running alone, I can feel them energizing me. By the way, I have about twenty years on all of them. It is a fact they won't let me forget, but I love them nonetheless.

My good friend, Alan, and I used to hit the tennis courts a few years ago. He would mercilessly beat up on me until it felt like my heart would burst. For some insane reason, I kept coming back for more. He pushed me to the edge. It didn't kill me, so maybe I'm stronger! Alan encouraged me to share some of my secrets for staying young and maintaining optimal health. I owe him dearly for that.

The younger generations at the gym where I work inspire me beyond belief. I want to be more like them, full of ideas, energy, dreams, boldness and enthusiasm. Some like to call me "old man" even though I am not that old, it would seem. However, I guess when you are in your 20s, a 50-plus year-old man might seem ancient.

Without my friends I would not be able to do my job and maintain my sanity. They push me to the brink and pull me back in good form. They are the main inspirations for **The 1st Aisle.**

Before moving forward, I should say some things about my history and formulation of my ideology. As a kid I grew up eating anything and everything. I especially loved soul food. Pancakes, sausage, eggs, toast and milk was my desired breakfast. There was nothing like fried chicken, spare ribs, candied yams and mac'n'cheese. On Thanksgiving I always got my full share of sweet potato pie and eggnog (spiked with whiskey when available). And junk food? Lots of weekends I rode my bike to Carvel's to get vanilla ice-cream on a sugar cone, after finishing off chili dogs at Father & Son's. A friend's father always had Peanut M&M's waiting for me when I would visit. It was hard to resist Sara Lee Chocolate Cake. I was relatively healthy and a good athlete, playing football, basketball and tennis. Sure, I got sick like everyone else with colds and the flu, but I was not aware that anything I was eating would cause health problems. I guess I was a typical kid growing up in Linden, New Jersey.

Then something happened in the mid-1980s. My late Aunt Pepsi introduced me to water fasting. The first time was rough, but I lasted three days. Then, in 1986, I decided to give up red meat to see what would happen. On New Year's Eve of 1987 I gave up chicken and the following New Year's Eve I gave up fish. Then I went to a Tony Robbins event. Tony said, "If you fed a baby calf milk from a supermarket, it would die." Little did I know I was venturing into veganism.

My transition to veganism was not to lose weight or overcome any illness. I just wanted to live a higher quality life. My thinking was that there must be a formula to keep me strong and healthy forever, so I started asking questions, reading books and going to presentations. Back then everyone thought I was delusional, as many still do now. But, I kept moving forward in my quest for more powerful information. My hunch was that the fruit and vegetable kingdom was the best place to start poking around, and off I went. It was the best move I've ever made.

During my transition, I began to feel better and look better. I was "pigging out" on broccoli, carrots and onions. I went to salad bars all the time. I ate all the advertised vegan food you could imagine. During holidays, especially Thanksgiving, dinner was collard greens, rice and mashed potatoes, but without turkey. Of course, my family thought I was crazy. My cousins would always ask, "Cuz, you still not eatin' meat?" After 29 years the answer is still no.

Luck struck me in the early '90s when a friend introduced me to Angelica Kitchen, the best vegan restaurant in Manhattan. After tasting the food there, I knew I could never turn back. I was shocked by what could be done without meat products as I became totally addicted to my newfound vegan cuisine.

Going vegan and striving to be a whole food plant-based eater has by far been my greatest achievement and greatest asset (*see Appendix A – My Day as a 1st Aisler*). It has kept me energized and vibrant. Many of the metabolic infirmities family, friends and clients are struggling with have not affected me at this point. Of course, I am working on delaying them for as long as possible. Thus far

I can do far more physically than most people I know and I'm always receiving compliments that I look 15 or more years younger than I am. My only dismay is that I have a hole in my afro and cannot get my hair to grow in. Obviously, life is far from perfect.

Since most people believe my physical results are superlative, it makes me perfectly suited to be a personal trainer. It's not a high-profile job, but most people are envious that I get to go to work in shorts and a tee shirt, which I love by the way. The jewel of my profession is that it has given me the opportunity to understand the knowledge that people have, as well as their misconceptions, about food, nutrition and healing. That said, during my sessions with clients, I always stress greater raw fruit and vegetable consumption. Beyond a shadow of a doubt, it is where youth begins and how strength can be maintained.

As a personal trainer, I am not a food scientist, nutritionist, herbalist, medical doctor or anything that takes a huge amount of "brain power." I greatly respect all those professions, but oftentimes technical expertise obscures the simplicity and power of nature. *The 1st Aisle* is not "dependent" upon science to be effective. Most "food science" appears to be highly questionable at best, obviated by the steady rise of metabolic diseases. *The 1st Aisle* is simply the perspectives of a personal trainer with 29 years of veganism and plant-based eating experience, combined with additional anecdotal and statistical information. That makes this work of art highly opinionated, but it is based on real-life results I have personally experienced or witnessed. My philosophy is that common sense always trumps science when it comes to food.

Many references to online material, as well as print material, are included in this book. There are those who will severely criticize online sources and cry, "You can't believe everything you read on the Internet." Well, as the average citizen, with limited scientific education and no letters after my name, I tend to rely on the Internet for information. As you read further, if some source seems questionable, take your time and fact check that source. Is the online information from the World Health Organization and United States Department of Agriculture faulty? Are the abstracts from PubMed.com biased and a waste of time to scour through? I cannot be certain, but we must begin our journey somewhere. Regardless, do not totally rely on any source for information on optimal health or wellbeing. As Ronald Reagan admonished us, "Trust, but verify." Keep in mind that reason and research are great weapons, but your best weapon is enlightenment through experience.

Lastly, my mission is to be the go-to personal trainer who deciphers all the nutritional information spinning in your head. There are way too many diet books with contrasting theories on what it takes to be healthy. Very few of us will read all the way through them, from start to finish. Therefore, my gut tells me that we need an intermediary to bridge the gap between the erudition of doctors, dieticians, food scientists and researchers, to the average citizen like you and me, who uses common sense and may know little to nothing about nutrition. The average citizen's time is fully occupied with putting food on the table, paying the rent and squeezing in time for relaxation. If you are in that same boat, clamoring for direction on what to eat, I'm giving you all I've got.

In the end, you will be the best judge of what works for you. My bottom line is simple: never argue with success. If something works and no harm is done to anyone, I will not argue against it, even if I do not believe in it. Have faith in your experience and the wisdom emanating from it. If you apply a suggestion from this book and you feel younger and more energized, that is all you really need to know to continue moving forward. The tendency may be to fight success because a new fad is sweeping the nation and you don't want to be left in the dust. If, however, application of a commonsense suggestion starts to improve the quality of your life, should it be ignored? I don't think so. Take it and run with it.

Introduction

America is in a state of crisis. The diseases associated with metabolic syndrome (heart disease, type 2 diabetes, high blood pressure, high cholesterol, obesity and cancer) are ravaging us. The World Health Organization predicts that by 2050 cancer rates will soar by 57%; and type 2 diabetes will jump from 1 in 8 people to 1 in 4.[1] Coupled with this is the lack of accessibility to healthcare, and the associated skyrocketing costs. Given the current economic climate, it's easy to go bankrupt just to stay alive.

The younger generations are never too fearful when these types of stats and potential disasters are thrown at them. They are bold and they do not break down as much as older folks do, so youth obviously has its advantages. But, assuming you're getting up there in age like me, and maybe you're breaking down too much to your liking, then it makes one wonder what it would be like to stay forever young. This book was written to satisfy that sense of wonderment. Its purpose is to stymie the effects of metabolic syndrome so we may maintain youth and vitality later in life. Tapping into the fountain of youth may sound unrealistic to most, but accepting it as a challenge is a decision I implore you to make. If you do so, you can decelerate the aging process, live an exceptional life filled with an

Metabolic Syndrome

5 risk factors that increase the likelihood of developing heart disease, cancer, diabetes, and stroke:

1. *Increased blood pressure*
2. *Increased blood sugar*
3. *Excess abdominal fat*
4. *High triglyceride levels*
5. *Low levels of good cholesterol (HDL)*

abundance of energy, and consequently experience much more joy. All you must do to meet the challenge is come to an understanding: nature has provided the resources for you to get the job done, through the power of plant-based eating.

Over the last eight years, as a personal trainer, I've conducted more than 10,000 hours of individual and group training sessions. During those training sessions I have learned much about the physical and mental pain many of us are grappling with—mostly due to living against nature—by consuming foods that don't agree with us metabolically. When my clients adopt food choice changes and enhancements that I recommend, mostly emanating from the first aisle of the supermarket, positive results begin to flow. Feelings of more energy and lightness are very common. Many are astonished at how easy the process is and how quickly it works. *The 1st Aisle* is here to link us to the source of what makes us stronger, better, more confident, wiser and ultimately, more content with who we are.

Originally this book was entitled "How to Stay Young Through the Power of Plant-Based Eating". When I told a friend of the title she scowled, "There's nuthin' wrong with growing old!" Another smart-alecky friend asked, "Oh yeah, how's that going for you?" Yes, Father Time is undefeated, but it's never been about defeating Father Time. It's about "influencing" Father Time so you may mature like a fine bottle of wine.

Introduction

We all want the experience and wisdom of aging, but we would all trade in a body rife with decay and malfunction for a new and improved model. When the knees crackle, the back stiffens, the blood pressure escalates, the vision blurs, the arteries corrode and the belly bulges, then it's not too pretty. Quite frankly, those physical "eventualities" of aging scare me beyond belief.

For the sake of full disclosure, **The 1st Aisle** is a message based on my two biggest fears: getting old and getting sick. More importantly, it is about

> *Nutritional excellence is the only real fountain of youth. — Joel Fuhrman,*

how I manage those fears through the first aisle of the grocery store. There's absolutely nothing wrong with the aging process, as it simply cannot be avoided. But getting old too quickly is not something to strive for. And, getting sick in many cases is avoidable, if we exercise discipline regarding what we eat. Therefore, if you share my fears, let's use them for motivation, not stultification. They should fuel us to push forward and search for answers. If we do not stay on top of our game and we become lazy, then aging and sickness will shackle us. We will become prisoners in our own bodies. Something tells me you do not want that.

Once, at a Thanksgiving dinner, a friend sarcastically replied to my fear of growing old, "Well, I've got news for you, there is nothing you can do about it. There's nothing to fear." Everyone looked at me like I was a fool, but I didn't feel the urge to engage in verbal fisticuffs at such a festive occasion. It would not have been a fair fight. She was my age, at least 30 pounds overweight, and in very suspect physical condition. However, I have got good news for her and for the listening world: there is something to fear, but there is also something you can do about it! There is always an action to take that could ameliorate your situation. Believe it or not, we can influence how we get old and how we get sick through exercise and eating. And, by the way, that friend asked me about eating tips later during the evening. Her grandiose statement of fearlessness was obviously a cover up. Apparently, she feared physical deterioration and accelerated aging as much as I did. I am pleased to say she took my recommendations to heart and she is doing quite well.

> *I have argued for years that we do not have a health care system in America. We have a disease-management system - one that depends on ruinously expensive drugs and surgeries that treat health conditions after they manifest rather than giving our citizens simple diet, lifestyle and therapeutic tools to keep them healthy.*
> *– Andrew Weil*

Accepting personal responsibility for our health and well-being is exactly what *The 1st Aisle* is all about. As of now, most of

America is at the mercy of the healthcare and pharmaceutical industries. We have relinquished control to entities that do not always have our best interests at heart. Far too often profit margin stands in the way of the pricelessness of healthy living. However, now is the perfect opportunity to wrest control from the healthcare and drug industries and begin the healing process. All we need is an empowering way to see and interpret food that relieves digestive stress, which, in turn, promotes the energy and resources needed to combat and defeat disease. *The 1st Aisle* is the empowering way that we can accomplish this goal.

The two pie charts that follow depict the objective of *The 1st Aisle*. The first is the Standard American Diet (SAD) from the United States Department of Agriculture Economic Research Service.[2] It is 88% processed and animal foods, which specializes in promoting digestive stress and depleting energy. It is an extremely effective eating philosophy at proliferating metabolic diseases such as cancer, high blood pressure, type 2 diabetes and high cholesterol.

Standard American Diet (SAD)

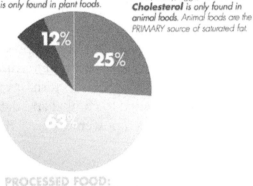

PLANT FOOD:
Vegetables, Fruits, Legumes,
Nuts & Seeds, Whole Grains
Fiber is only found in plant foods.

ANIMAL FOOD:
Meat, Dairy, Eggs, Fish, Seafood
Cholesterol is only found in
animal foods. Animal foods are the
PRIMARY source of saturated fat.

12%

25%

63%

PROCESSED FOOD:
Added Fats & Oils, Sugars, Refined Grains

The next pie chart is Raw Energy Vitality (REV), composed of 75% plant-based foods. It reduces digestive stress and increases energy in a safe and efficient manner. Although I am a staunch plant-based food advocate, the initial objective is not to immediately jump into a first aisle eating style. The thought of that induces stress in most omnivores and they immediately reject the idea. The decision to go whole food plant-based can be made once you are more familiar with the power of plant foods. With that in mind, there are some animal products (15%) and "fun" foods (10%) that may be consumed.

Raw Energy Vitality

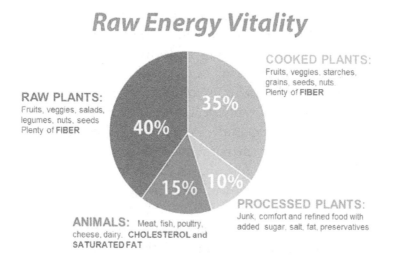

RAW PLANTS:
Fruits, veggies, salads,
legumes, nuts, seeds
Plenty of **FIBER**

COOKED PLANTS:
Fruits, veggies, starches,
grains, seeds, nuts.
Plenty of **FIBER**

35%

40%

15% 10%

ANIMALS: Meat, fish, poultry,
cheese, dairy. **CHOLESTEROL and
SATURATED FAT**

PROCESSED PLANTS:
Junk, comfort and refined food with
added sugar, salt, fat, preservatives

My belief is REV will eradicate 90% of our metabolic health issues. All you must do is consume a combination of 75% raw and cooked fruits and veggies. It is the safest way to energize your body for maximum healing and maximum performance.

The only way to know if REV works is to try it. If you do, experience tells me you'll love it. When your weight drops, your cholesterol drops, your blood pressure drops, your skin clears up, your energy elevates, and your positive attitude becomes infectious, you will feel unstoppable. The only question left is how to implement REV, which will be answered in the subsequent chapters.

Dare I say that, in 2018, we are at the beginning of a plant-based evolution in which REV will play a vital role. It has taken quite some time to get this evolution in motion because plant-based eating has a serious public relations issue: most people do not believe plants contain enough protein to make them big and strong, assuming they contain any protein at all. Of course, we all know how much we need the vitamins and minerals from plants, but protein translates into physical power in the minds of most Americans. Consequently, Americans are having a love affair with it and the mere mention of "protein" can boost product sales. To top it off, protein is inextricably linked to animal products through savvy marketing and advertising. That said, we would also be foolish to underestimate the emotional attachments many people have to meat, cheese and milk. Although there is strong evidence that vegetables contain sufficient amounts of protein, and even higher quality protein than animal products, it is sacrilegious for many people to hear that. Therefore, getting them to consume more plant-based food is an extremely hard sell.

However, to the rescue come some of the world's greatest heroes and role models: professional athletes! They are now proving that you can consume a preponderance of plant-based foods, eating little to no animal products, and perform at the highest level. More importantly, they are going public with their affinity for plant-based eating. Back in the 1980s and '90s, Carl Lewis won nine Olympic gold medals in track and field and was the fastest man in the world. He was deemed "World Athlete of the Century" by the International Association of Athletics Federations; "Sportsman of the Century" by the

International Olympic Committee; and "Greatest U.S. Olympian of the Century" by Sports Illustrated.[3] Carl Lewis professed that his plant-based/vegan lifestyle helped him perform at his best in 1990 at 30 years of age.[4] During his dominant years, however, metabolic diseases were not raging as they are now, nor were there opportunities such as searching the Internet in order to gather information or promote plant-based ideologies. About that same time, while I was starting a vegan lifestyle, I heard nothing about Carl Lewis' adoration for veganism in the media.

Fast-forward 28 years to 2018. The playing field is quite different. Metabolic syndrome is wreaking havoc and professional athletes have Twitter, Facebook, YouTube plus a bevy of other outlets at their fingertips to get information to the public instantaneously. If actors, singers and other entertainers were to promote plant-based eating, they could easily be ignored, or considered eccentric or quirky. But professional athletes are the emblems of superior masculine and feminine vitality and power. They are envied beyond belief. Many are international heroes and are paid unbelievable amounts of money for playing games on a field. With the clout professional athletes have, combined with Madison Avenue savvy, they can easily sway public opinion and take the plant-based evolution to soaring heights.

Tom Brady, quarterback for the New England Patriots, is a prime example of a superhero athlete. Brady attributes his long tenure in the National Football League to plant-based eating and a disciplined exercise regimen. Currently, he's the oldest quarterback in the NFL and will most likely retire as the greatest football player of all time. Although he has not committed publicly to going whole food plant-based (supposedly he eats small amounts of lean meat, but is vegan during parts of the year), he's playing at MVP levels into his 40s, something unheard of in the NFL. He and his wife, supermodel Gisele Bündchen, are the world's premier plant-based eating couple in the realm of sports. To the delight of plant-based advocates, Tom is using his fame and stature to promote his own signature brand of plant-based foods—TB12 Performance Meals—through the home delivery service The Purple Carrot. Kudos to Tom for taking it a step further by railing against the processed food industries, calling Coca-Cola poison for kids and implying that Frosted Flakes is not food.[5]

In 2011, Venus Williams, superstar and seven-time grand slam champion, was diagnosed with Sjögren's syndrome. It is an autoimmune disease where the mucous membranes and moisture-secreting glands of the eyes and mouth are affected, resulting in decreased tears and saliva. The condition often accompanies rheumatoid arthritis and lupus. Other symptoms are joint pain, swelling, dry skin, stiffness and prolonged fatigue. Sjögren's syndrome could have ended Venus' tennis career and destroyed the quality of her life. But, Venus took serious action by adopting a plant-based eating style to solve the problem. As she says, "I started for health reasons. I was diagnosed with an autoimmune disease, and I wanted to maintain my performance on the court. Once I started I fell in love with the concept of fueling your body in the best way possible. Not only does it help me on the court, but I feel like I'm doing the right thing for me. I literally couldn't play tennis anymore, so it really changed my life."[6] She has been wildly successful with her eating regimen and has remained one of the top female athletes in the world. At 37 years of age, she is also the oldest player on the ladies' tennis tour.

The most compelling sign that we have entered a plant-based evolution might be found with the Boston Celtics all-star point guard, Kyrie Irving. His heroic play won the NBA championship for the Cleveland Cavaliers in 2016, but Kyrie wanted more from himself physically. Then something seismic happened to the delight of the plant-based world in 2017. In the article *The Secret (But Healthy!) Diet Powering Kyrie and the NBA*, BleacherReport.com reported, "After a preseason game on ESPN, Irving announced something intriguing to Chauncey Billups and the NBA Countdown crew, who noticed how much...thinner he looked: 'Been on more of a plant-based diet, getting away from the animals and all that,' Irving told the broadcast team. 'I had to get away from that. So my energy is up; my body feels amazing.'"[7] It was an astonishing public statement to make, especially considering the meat based world we live in. It is the first time I have heard a top tier athlete advocate avoiding meat products gave him more energy!

However, there was an even more provocative episode signaling the beginning of the plant-based evolution. On

Christmas Day, Nike gave us a precious gift: a commercial featuring Kyrie Irving and his basketball wizardry. At the end of an amazing dribbling display, Kyrie is asked by New England Patriots tight end Rob Gronkowski, "How'd you do that?" Kyrie's response, "Simple. Plant-based diet."[8] The significance of that response cannot be underestimated. A top-tier athlete, sponsored by the biggest selling shoe brand of the NBA, espousing a plant-based diet? It's incredible. Kids and adults may see it and consider plant-based eating a viable alternative, especially if you want to be in tip-top physical condition and succeed at the highest professional level. It is a well-defined signal that things are changing for the better.

There are many other athletes involved in the plant-based evolution we have entered. Tennis superstar Novak Djokovic, winner of 12 Grand Slams, opened a vegan restaurant in Monte Carlo, Eqvita, in 2016. USAToday.com reported that 10 players on the Tennessee Titans football team went vegan during the 2017 season.[9] One of the best ultramarathoners in the world, Scott Jurek, has been vegan for the last 17 years and he has won more than 20 major races. The list of those eschewing animal products goes on and on. Hopefully they will carry the torch proudly, rescue us from metabolic syndrome and keep us young for a long time.

Lastly, for those who know me well, what follows may be shocking: I have freed myself from the bondage of "veganism." Veganism does not accurately depict what

The 1st Aisle truly involves. It suggests that giving up animal products is the panacea for the health woes of the world. That philosophy is far from the truth. I have tried all types of vegan foods, but most of what I have sampled appears to be "processed" vegan food that I consider garbage. Vegan food scientists are always concocting ways to imitate meat products that may be just as dangerous as any other type of processed food, although what they create may taste great. Of course, adopting veganism is the greatest thing in the world because of its ripple effects on the environment, economy and animal rights. But it is not beneficial for maximal health when it is processed with chemicals. Consequently, many people have not been pleased with their results and have become very disenchanted with veganism. Consuming too much processed food—regardless of its origin—is always a dangerous proposition.

Ironically, as a personal trainer, my first two clients, in 2010, were both "vegan" gentleman. The first was 6'2" tall and weighed about 300 pounds. He thoroughly enjoyed all forms of processed vegan food. When we first met he said, "I'm a vegan too, but as you can see I eat a lot of carbs!" The second gentleman was an inch taller, but only about 160 pounds. He would get on the treadmill and run like the wind, pump iron and do lots of core work, but he exercised restraint with processed foods and ate predominantly from the first aisle. Two gentlemen with similar stature who did not eat meat products, but each produced totally different results, all because of fresh produce consumption. By the way, I prefer my second client's results.

Since I no longer consider myself a vegan, what am I? I believe in eating plant-based food, but a lot of it is junk food vegan, so I eat very little of it. My greatest desire is benefitting from the powerful results that eating from the first aisle will certainly give me. Then I can help my clients get superior results, after I have already done the research and testing on myself. I am somewhere between vegan and whole food plant-based, therefore I simply refer to myself as a *1st Aisler* regarding my eating style (*see Appendix A – My Day as a 1st Aisler*). The sole objective of a *1st Aisler* is to move as close to whole food plant-based eating as possible for maximum physical results. There are no hard and fast rules, just an ideal to strive for, but there is room for flexibility as you must find what fits your lifestyle. Regardless of your individual choice of food, if you allow the first aisle to become your sanctuary, you will be amazed by the results. Philosophically I am a Resultatarian (*see Appendix B – The Age of the Resultatarian*), because it is all about results. After reading this book, you will be a Resultatarian too!

The 1st Aisle will play a part in the whole food plant-based evolution by opening the door to greater wisdom regarding what to eat. Above all else, it is focused on getting you to take immediate action. The "action" step is where we are stumbling in America. We have all the knowledge and information imaginable. It is literally right at our fingertips. We are inundated with facts, figures and studies, yet none of that gives us a step-by-step process to get the job done. You now have that process in your hands.

Meet you in the first aisle!

First, nutrition is the master key to human health. Second, what most of us think of as proper nutrition—isn't.

T. Colin Campbell, MD

The 1st Aisle Philosophy for Results

To embrace a first aisle eating style, we need a new perspective regarding aging, health, food and life. In the United States our viewpoints are strongly based on science, facts and statistics, or so we think. We have the best doctors, nutritionists and statisticians in the world and we heavily rely on them for guidance. As soon as they release the "latest study, " the media is all over it. We devour the knowledge—mostly headlines—and take it for granted that what is said is gospel.

For instance, until just recently eggs were considered somewhat hazardous in terms of heart health. For more than 50 years, doctors told us to cut down on egg consumption due to the link between high cholesterol levels and eventual heart disease. But, Americans love eggs. According to the American Egg Board (AEB), the "Incredible, Edible Egg" per capita consumption was 267 eggs in 2016.[10] Most people cannot imagine breakfast without them. The food industry adds them to all types of processed food for flavor and protein. (I've had many heated discussions regarding cakes needing eggs to rise; this, of course, is not true.) Then a new study comes out in 2013, and the United States Dietary Guidelines changed. High cholesterol levels in eggs are no longer considered dangerous to your health.[11] The media is giddy about the latest news. They pass it on to the public, and very few question the new guidelines. Thank the man upstairs we have the latest scientific information which confirms what we want to hear: we can get the party started and eat eggs with reckless abandon. What a relief!

Hold on! Where did this "latest scientific information" come from? We're told that doctors from Harvard concur, so it must be true. *The Washington Post, New York Times* and every major media outlet is reporting it, so the sources must be credible. Yet, let's dig a little deeper. The information that the U.S. Dietary Guidelines Advisory Committee (USDGAC) relied on to draw the conclusions comes predominantly from the egg industry, according to Neal Barnard, M.D., President of the Physicians Committee for Responsible Medicine (PCRM).[12] Of course, that makes the USDGAC's conclusions highly suspect since the egg industry has a vested interest in selling eggs. Dr. Barnard also adds that there is a money trail to prove it.

> *People love to hear good news about their bad habits. —*
> *John McDougall, MD*

The question is whose information should we follow? It is possible that Dr. Barnard and the PCRM are just a bunch of rogue physicians with weird theories about eating fruits and veggies. On the other hand, the USDGAC is whispering sweet nothings about the virtues of eggs in our ears. Looks like the USDGAC is a winner! But, the real issue is, as Americans, we've brainwashed ourselves to believe that "experts" have the information we need regarding healthy eating. Furthermore, we have convinced ourselves that we are helpless without them.

Now is the time for a new vantage point regarding what we think about food and nutrition. If we are lucid and focused, we will see a clear path to assume responsibility for our health and thwart metabolic diseases before they consume us. Fortunately, all the input and information we need is at our fingertips, craving to be accessed and put into action. It all begins with *The 1st Aisle Philosophy*.

The 1st Aisle Philosophy

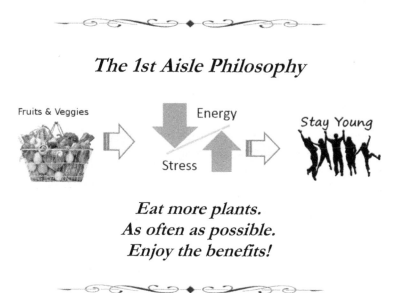

Fruits & Veggies

Energy

Stress

Stay Young

Eat more plants.
As often as possible.
Enjoy the benefits!

If we simply implant *The 1st Aisle Philosophy* in our minds, most of our metabolic problems begin to dissipate. To take it a step further: *the greater the percentage of food we eat from The 1st Aisle, the younger and healthier we will be.* It is not esoteric, nor does it require an advanced degree to understand. You do not need to know anything about nutrition to benefit from it. There are no magic pills to pop, nor is there a financial investment to be made. All you need to be aware of is that the first aisle of the grocery store is usually the fresh produce aisle. It is where all the vitamins and minerals hang out in their natural form. More importantly, it is the aisle that you and I must completely embrace, if we are truly interested in healthy living and staying young.

To bring deeper meaning to *The 1st Aisle Philosophy*, we must be on the same page regarding words and terms we use to define health and vitality.

Aging vs. "Olding"

Aging is the process of moving through time, while "olding" is the process of losing energy over time, and it is "olding" that accelerates your biological age (how old your body is, regardless of your chronological age). Therefore, you may be 50 years of age, but you can feel like 75 years old.

Let's look at the profiles of two middle-aged men:

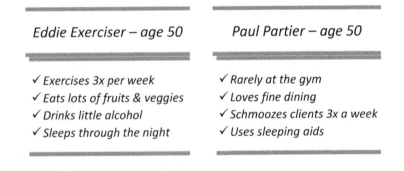

Eddie Exerciser – age 50	*Paul Partier – age 50*
✓ Exercises 3x per week	✓ Rarely at the gym
✓ Eats lots of fruits & veggies	✓ Loves fine dining
✓ Drinks little alcohol	✓ Schmoozes clients 3x a week
✓ Sleeps through the night	✓ Uses sleeping aids

Intuitively, which one would you guess looks older? I'd bet my last nickel you would pick Paul Partier. Why? Because you sense that his lifestyle is flooded by toxicity and stress, based on his profile. In your experience, you surely remember that being a party animal can wear you down quickly. To the contrary, you sense that Eddie Exerciser's lifestyle suppresses toxicity. You know that when you exercise and eat well, you feel fantastic. Both gentlemen are the same chronological age, but Paul Partier is "olding" faster than Eddie Exerciser, due to a toxic lifestyle.

Visualize a classic car which has been well maintained by its owner when thinking of age. It looks pristine and rides like a charm, only because the owner took exquisite care of it for a long time. However, many people travel in the opposite direction. Their cars are broken down quite often due to rugged abuse. Your body is your vehicle. You are the mechanic and you are the driver.

The biggest difference between those two gentlemen is something you cannot see on the outside: metabolic energy. Metabolic energy is the energy needed to efficiently digest food and use its nutrients to fight disease, promote growth and enhance physical and mental performance. You may sense that Eddie has it in abundance, while Paul does not, due to their respective lifestyle choices. Staying young is about harnessing energy and burning it efficiently through the power of plant-based eating. As a personal trainer I commonly see a 25-year gap in the energy and performance levels of two people who are the same age. I have a client, Pete, who is 60 years of age. He has been running since his college years and can easily outrun many 30-year-olds. I have another client the same age that neglected his body for the last 20 years. Consequently, he moves like he's 75 years old. Getting out of the bed in the morning is often a challenge. It almost brings tears to my eyes to work with him. Of course, that gap in energy and performance level greatly impacts quality of life. The gap is not necessarily good versus bad, it is purely the manifestation of how one chooses to live their life.

Olding is a Gradual Process

Think of "olding" as rowing a boat across a lake. As you row, your boat goes through wear and tear and water leaks in. Eventually, the leaks become overwhelming, so you take time away from rowing to make some repairs. You start rowing again, but it is more difficult since you have exhausted energy and time.

Maybe you have experienced something similar as you move through life and a health issue suddenly arises, demanding your attention. Early on you do not pay much attention to it because you were young and powerful. It may have annoyed you a bit, but it did not impact your quality of life. Eventually the health issue became overpowering as your body was forced to divert energy to heal. You then had to bail out the toxicity and plug up the holes in your body using medical professionals and prescription drugs. As you recovered you began to move forward again, but now at a slower rate. Permanent damage may have been done. You have grown older and there may be lingering effects of toxicity. You may even feel 20 years older.

In many cases "olding" is a gradual process of not paying attention to the obvious. We are all guilty of overlooking health-related issues. We tend to procrastinate when they pop up. Oftentimes we deny our health is in jeopardy. Before you know it, middle age hits at 40 and you look and feel like you are 60.

Does "Olding" Run in the Family?

Over the course of time we accept a certain status quo for "olding", consequently we are not pressed to take immediate action when our bodies revolt against us. We misunderstand and adopt the belief that metabolic maladies, such as diabetes, obesity and heart disease, are part of the "olding" process. Many believe those diseases are simply inevitable. Your mother has high blood pressure, your father has diabetes and so you incorrectly presume you will fall prey to them too. It just runs in the family!

One of the premises of this book is that genetics can be irrelevant in many instances. The notion that genetics is destiny dwells in the mind of too many people. That way of thinking must be obliterated

> *Genetics loads the gun; lifestyle pulls the trigger. – Caldwell Esselstyn, MD*

to embrace the full power of plant-based eating. What matters is how you mitigate or overcome any genetic predisposition you may have—and it all begins with a sense of urgency. The healing process starts with a new and improved eating philosophy, based on an enhanced vision of one's self. It must be clearly understood that the person staring at you in the mirror is in control of what goes in your mouth. If that person makes the best choices, 95% of metabolic problems go away. There is no need to be trapped by metabolic diseases. What runs in your family does not have to run over you.

Mentality vs. Reality

One's concept of the word "young" has a lot to do with performance level and overall health, but it is mainly due to mentality. Of course, genes do play a significant part, but genes are simply the dimensions of the playing field. How the game is played determines your destiny. When your body is supplied with the type of food meant for it, you will maintain higher levels of energy, overcome your genetic shortcomings and be at your best. You will not easily succumb to the characteristics of "olding". Those characteristics many would deem as part of the "aging process." I would agree, to an extent. The real question is the rate at which those characteristics

> **"Olding" Characteristics**
>
> Lack of energy
> Lack of stamina
> Lack of flexibility
> Muscle atrophy
> Stiffness
> Loss of posture
> Loss of balance
> Metabolic diseases

"overwhelm" the body. The slower the rate, the younger you will be for an extended period of time.

Once I was speaking with a gentleman who was battling prostate cancer and deciding whether to get his prostate removed. He told me the disease was part of the aging process and nothing could be done about it. At age 69 was he too young for his prostate to be compromised to the point where it had to be removed? There is no way to know, but for the entirety of his life he never paid attention to the first aisle of the supermarket. Is it possible the severity of his situation could have been mitigated to some degree, with a heightened awareness of the power of plant-based food and exercise? We certainly cannot prove it, but something tells me there would have been a difference. Change the mentality and you can change the man.

Good Food vs. Bad Food

So, now that you know the premise of **_The 1st Aisle_**, this section may seem contradictory or odd, but there are no good foods, nor are there any bad foods. Good and bad are purely judgments and nothing else. The fact is, food is either beneficial or detrimental, based on your situation. If you're starving on a deserted island and someone drops donuts and pizza from an airplane, something tells me you're going to eat it and enjoy it. And, you will probably get good results from those foods compared to not eating at all. You need energy to live and even the worst foods give you some energy. However, if you have access to fresh fruits and veggies and you choose pizza and donuts, relatively speaking, they would be bad for you. What matters most is what a particular food can do for you at any particular moment. The *Standard American Diet Food Funnel* shows us the problem we have and what it produces:

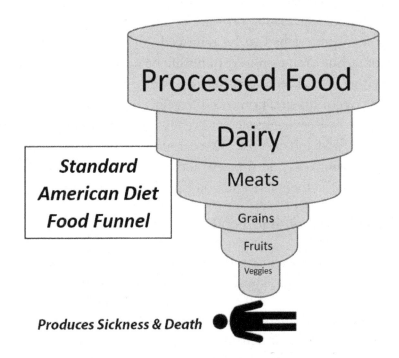

Most of what goes in the funnel is processed food. The least of what goes in are fresh veggies, which we need the most to be metabolically vibrant. I have had many debates on that point, but your body craves veggies and fruits. It thrives when they are poured into your body in abundance.

All we must do is flip the food proportions and we have *The 1st Aisle Food Funnel*, a recipe for success!

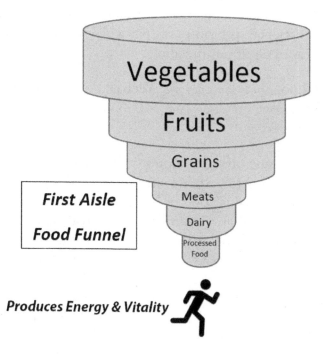

The Nutrient Battle

Too much time and energy is wasted analyzing nutrients to justify which foods should be praised or condemned. For example, if a certain food contains a higher percentage of protein, most would assume it builds muscle, therefore it must be good for you. But, what if that same food had been shown to accelerate cancer growth? Does packing on extra muscle make up for the cancerous effects? That is for you to decide. If a certain food contains a higher percentage of fat, the assumption is that it is bad for you. However, certain types of fat are critical for optimal metabolic functioning. The problem arises when some "new" science promotes a particular nutrient as the panacea for all of our metabolic woes.

In the book, *In Defense of Food*, Michael Pollan warns us that we are now in the Age of Nutritionism.[13] It is characterized by:

1. Focusing on consumption of nutrients, not foods.
2. The need for experts with specialized knowledge to tell us what is good or bad to eat.
3. A battle of good nutrients versus bad nutrients.
4. Assuming the main reason for eating is nutrient value and health.

Doctors, nutritionists, scientists and engineers are far more erudite than the average person. Yet, with their specialized knowledge, metabolic syndrome is raging out of control. One issue that Pollan identifies is that a food is not the sum of its nutrient parts. If we break down an orange into all its nutrient parts, for some reason we cannot put those nutrients back together again and create an orange. Furthermore, we cannot add nutrients to a food and improve it.

The food industry has been working on improving food for many years, through food "fortification," and it is a daunting proposition. In fact, the World Health

Organization and the Food and Agricultural Organization of the United Nations have produced the *Guidelines on Food Fortification with Micronutrients[14]*, supported through funding from the Global Alliance for Improved Nutrition (GAIN). It's 300-plus pages of recommendations regarding what should and shouldn't be done to food. Yet, with all the directives and knowledge it contains, cancer, obesity and type 2 diabetes rates are projected to climb. It appears that the recommendations accomplish one thing: the addition of nutrients into inferior food products, which are usually tasteless, high in calories, packaged, mass produced and, of course, low in nutrients. Those inferior food products are affectionately known as "junk food" or "empty-calorie food." No amount of food fortification will strengthen them.

We have been dropped smack dab in the middle of a nutrient battle. Many of us will be casualties of war through eating foods we know are killing us. Others will be taken out by friendly fire through eating foods we are conditioned to believe are good for us. As of 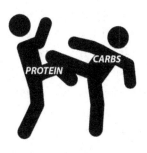 this writing, it seems to be carbs versus protein; omega-3 versus omega-6; probiotics versus antibiotics. No one knows who the victor will be because we're waiting for the latest study to give us direction. It's a complete mess and bodies are dropping senselessly. We must get out of the crosshairs and find refuge.

A Safe Haven

Amidst all the nutrition-induced chaos, the safest place to retreat is the first aisle of the grocery store. That is where our efforts must begin for healthy living and youthful exuberance. Our focus should not be on consuming individual nutrients or minerals with hoped for results. We must concentrate on eating whole foods that produce positive results. Doing it the latter way we do not have to be scientific genii to figure out what to eat.

All over the world people eat different foods, based on culture and geography. In America we have access to all types of food because we are blessed with a high standard of living. With what we have available, we could produce a wide range of metabolic results. Therefore, it is highly advisable to focus on getting the results that you want, then determining which eating style and foods will produce that result. In my experience and through client observations, focusing on plant-based foods will yield nothing but positive results. When you venture outside of the first aisle of the grocery store to satisfy your palate—except for water, grains, beans and rice—danger is lurking around the corner. All the lower levels of The 1st Aisle *Food Funnel* come into play and hell breaks loose.

Do the Right Thing!

Results are the name of the game; make no mistake about it. I knew a guy at the gym who I thought looked fabulous.

He ate all the fruits and veggies and did all the right things, yet he was unhappy with his results. There was another guy I thought needed some serious work. His eating philosophy was anything goes and it showed in the shape of his body. I vehemently disagreed with what he decided to eat, but he appeared to be as happy as could be. Obviously those two gentlemen had different expectations and desires. This poses the question—was each getting the results he wanted in terms of health, based on the foods each had chosen?

The "all the right thingers" and the "anything goers" raise a few issues. First, most of those who do "all the right things" regarding food choices are subject to what they "think" is right. Unfortunately, most of what they think is right comes from highly questionable sources. For example, I've seen many milk advertisements propagating the benefits of protein and calcium in their dairy products. After watching those commercials, one might unequivocally believe that milk is the best thing in the world to drink. Yet, deeper research may not support the advertisers' claims. Of course, we need protein and calcium, but is milk the best source for them? Many would say absolutely not and there's a lot of science to support this claim.[15]

Second, for many people claiming to do "all the right things," it can produce tons of stress and confusion. They food shop based on all the latest research. They pull out the magnifying glass and scrutinize every nutrition label. They buy organic products at the fanciest markets. They have the best allergists, cardiologists and internists money can buy. Yet many of them are in highly suspect physical condition. They suffer from orthorexia nervosa, an unhealthy obsession with healthy eating. Consequently, they are sick way too much and flip-flop from one food fad to the next, hoping to find "the cure" for their physical infirmities. Yes, it is possible they are genetically inferior with weaker immune systems, but that's usually not the reason for their woes. The real deal is what they think is the "right" thing to do is what has become popular, not that which produces superior metabolic results. They cannot think independently so they're always subject to what the media deems to be good or bad.

> *Poor nutrition trumps tobacco, alcohol, and sedentary lifestyles as the primary cause of the development of chronic illnesses. We cannot ignore the reality that what we eat is totally within our control, and our choices are what determine the level of risk we have of becoming ill. —* Baxter Montgomery, MD

Third, how we measure results could be problematic. Working in a gym I see lots of patrons consuming all types of colorful energy and protein drinks. Many of those who consume those liquids get the results they want: they're packing on muscle at an accelerated rate. However, over the long term, are they destined for tragedy? Dare I say that all those concoctions are dangerous and haven't been researched thoroughly. The long-term effects are mysterious, although we do know that excessive protein causes myriad problems.

Lastly, for those with whom I disagree regarding the "anything goes" eating style, are they truly happy with their physical appearances? They go on and on about all the "good tasting" food they eat. They just "love" to eat and cannot understand how gastronomic discipline may be beneficial. Most are overweight and/or unhealthy and don't seem at all concerned about it. But, if you catch them in a moment of complete candor, oftentimes you'll find that they're not so happy at all. They can be the life of the party, laughing and carousing all night long, but there always seems to be melancholy lurking once the party is over.

Once, after a night of drinking and partying, a dear friend had an emotional breakdown. She's always been known to flaunt her sexuality and exude extreme confidence, so it appeared that her weight gain didn't bother her at all. However, after the party, she began crying and confessing. She was completely distraught about being 40-pounds overweight, its health complications and how it made her look. All the while I thought she was happy the way she was. Since that time, after coming to know and train many clients at the gym, I've found that no one is happy with being overweight and out of shape. They may appear happy on the outside, but inside they're struggling. That said, the "anything goes" eating philosophy must be thrown in the trash.

Race to the Finish Line

There is a "race" going on which most of us are completely unaware of: heartbeats versus energy. Let's assume you are born with a definite number of heartbeats over the course of your life, determined by your genes. Regardless of what you do, you cannot increase your allotment. To the contrary, you can subtract from your allotment of heartbeats over your lifetime. Factors that downgrade that allotment include environmental toxins, drugs, physical trauma, accidents, negative emotions and inactivity, all of which put stress on the body. However, now is the time to focus on the downgrading factor you have the most control over: the food you choose to eat. By far, it is the most influential component of maintaining energy and staying young.

If your heartbeats are downgraded due to ill-advised food choices, two things could happen. Obviously, you may live a shorter life and the life you live may not be as fruitful. Most likely you will suffer from a variety and/or severity of metabolic diseases. The "race" is to reach your allotment of heartbeats (the end of your life) maximally energized, before toxicity (disease) consumes you. Essentially you want to die in good health.

Imagine that you are running a marathon throughout your life and the finish line is far in the distance, but the Grim Reaper is hot on your tail. If you are fast and agile the Grim Reaper does not have a chance to catch you. You'll break the tape and go out on top. But, if you lack energy, he'll chop away at you, breaking you down piece by piece. It takes metabolic energy to outrun the toxic blows of the Grim Reaper because disease is the name of his game.

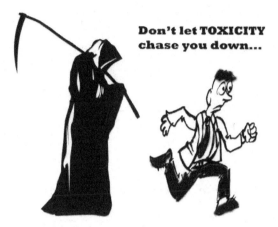

Don't let TOXICITY chase you down...

How we arrive at death tells the story of how we have lived. Living a life riddled with toxicity will be laborious and painful, but it can be avoided. The following graph will help tell the story.

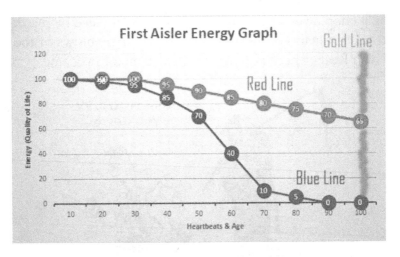

(This graph is for illustrative purposes only.)

The gold vertical line represents your maximum number of heartbeats. If you reach the gold vertical line, the question is *how* you reach it? It could be in grand style or beset by stress and related diseases.

The red line represents the ideal life and it is the maximum amount of energy for you to have, based on genetics. Understand that no one reaches the maximum because no one is perfect, although it is something to shoot for. While the red line is on a downward path, it is a gradual decline of energy, resulting from aging. It represents health and vibrancy, without the devastation of disease ravaging the body. Yes, you will manifest diseases and infirmities on the red line because you can't totally escape toxicity. However, toxicity can be mitigated so it only throws you off course a bit. By staying as close to the red line as possible, you will have the maximum energy necessary to combat metabolic diseases so you will not be taken out prematurely.

The blue line represents the energy level of the average person. It starts high, the same as the red line, but it quickly diverges. Between 30 to 40 years of age it begins to dip dramatically. Around 50 it plummets downward due to digestive stress. Near 70 it begins to level off where you only have enough energy to hang on, without exerting yourself too much. Eventually the blue line person dies prematurely between ages 70 to 80, as he is consumed and ravaged by metabolic diseases. Excessive toxicity accelerates the drastic drop in energy represented by the blue line.

As you can see, there is a wide energy gap between the red and blue lines that needs to be closed. All of us will fall below the red line since we're not perfect, but the closer we get to it energy-wise, the younger we will be. It is purely a quality of life issue. The goal is to run out of heartbeats while your energy level is high. As oxymoronic as it sounds, the ideal life is to die in good health. After that final heartbeat has struck, people will say about you, "I just saw him yesterday and he looked fabulous!" You simply ran out of heartbeats and went out as a champion.

A plant-based eating style will help you find a superior way to live. It is a philosophy of hope and inspiration. It is a way to fuse the lifestyle you want with the physical presence that you deserve. If you hang around in that first aisle long enough, it is a surefire guarantee that you will find the answers you've been hoping for. Eventually you'll build momentum toward a spectacular life filled with youthful exuberance!

The idea is to die young as late as possible. – Ashley Montagu

Raw Energy Vitality (REV)

Since 1989 I've been convinced that plant-based eating is the primary reason for the boost in my energy level. Furthermore, I believe that eating a higher percentage of raw fruits and veggies is the key to superior metabolic functioning. That realization prompted me to create a corporate presentation entitled *Raw Energy Vitality*.

It's All About Raw Energy

Raw Energy Vitality (REV) began as step-by-step process for my clients to transition to a first aisle eating style. With that eating style they have better workouts, get better results and appear to be much happier. That is all I ask for as a personal trainer. We already eat plenty of cooked food in America and much of it is highly processed, which fuels metabolic syndrome. The hurdle is that most people need to be cajoled into eating greater quantities of raw fruits and veggies. This is especially true of our kids who always want the fun foods they see in commercials. To keep them happy and quiet we appease them with food that is driving metabolic syndrome through the roof. We do not realize the degree to which we're hurting ourselves and future generations. This must be changed immediately.

Currently, the nutrition/dietary universe is littered with sinkholes and landmines. There are way too many theories and studies to scour through. Every few years we're seduced by the latest dietary fad with scientific studies to support it. And, to keep you chasing your tail, you can also find evidence to discredit the latest dietary fad. No one is quite sure if the dieticians, researchers, journalists, food manufacturers, pharmaceutical companies and food

> *The fad diets that many Americans are on are perfect if you want to be hungry all the time and miserable.*
> *— Nathan Pritikin*

scientists we rely upon for guidance are about healing or profiting. Given how metabolic syndrome is raging out of control, it appears that making money is at the root of the nutritional chaos we're drowning in. But, my clients want accurate information and answers immediately. Many are sick and tired of being sick and tired and they can't take it anymore. Therefore, the question arises: Is there a way to produce more energy, defeat the battle of the bulge and live a life of supreme physical fitness that we can all agree upon? Surely there must be a common nutritional thread to get us going in the right direction. REV is that common thread.

Going Once, Going Twice...Sold!

The issue we face is the food we desire so zealously is what we've been "sold" on. The food producers and advertisers are highly skilled. They know what buttons to press to get you to buy their products. With the right mixture of salt, fat and sugar, along with sexy imagery and celebrity endorsements, the average American can be seduced into consuming anything without question. Admittedly whole, plant-based food does not have the type of sex appeal processed food has to make you crave it because no one has dressed it up and made it pretty. Whether it is raw or cooked, plant-based food tastes better than processed food, but this is not a focus of food producers. They do not profit from it, so it is basically ignored.

Plant-based food is not a significant part of the mainstream social fabric. You go out with your friends and they want something quick, easy and accessible, which is the hallmark of highly processed food. Over time you start to pick up a couple of pounds in the wrong places, but everybody does, so who cares? Lo and behold, you're losing the battle of the bulge. America is just getting bigger, fatter and sicker, purely based on harmful food choices. The SAD (Standard American Diet) is surely not the answer, while solely eating plant-based food "appears" to be too extreme for most. This makes the mission of REV more challenging—or dare I say more exciting.

Have you ever wondered that there are no negative health consequences of eating fresh fruits or veggies? Setting aside allergies and autoimmune diseases (e.g. inflammatory bowel disease), they are not inherently detrimental to your health. For example, you probably never heard that oranges are bad for you because they contain too much vitamin C or calcium. But, on the flipside, we can find tons of information to condemn meat, dairy and processed food. They are linked to obesity, cancer, high cholesterol, etcetera, yet the advertisers tout the benefits of them.

According to the CDC, in 1960 the Average American male weighed 166 lbs. In 2015 the Average American male weighed 195 lbs.

With plant foods being beneficial and non-plant foods being detrimental, the answer becomes glaringly obvious: eat a higher percentage of fruits and veggies. Furthermore, the higher the percentage, the better off you will be. It seems obvious, but very few are taking that route. All information points out that greater fruit and vegetable consumption reduces rates of disease. Focusing on that singular point is the common thread amongst most of the dietary theories. It is the game changer we need and the focus of REV.

Is It Really as Simple as Eating More Veggies?

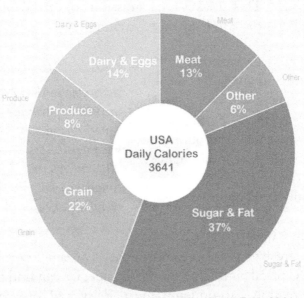

National Geographic - What the World Eats, 2011

In 2011, only 8% of calories of the average American's diet were obtained from fruits and vegetables, according to *National Geographic*, based on research from the Food and Agriculture Organization of the United Nations.[16] And, to add insult to injury, included in the fruits and vegetables category are potato chips and French fries, which obviously don't help the cause. Where has that eating style guided us? Into a deepening pit of metabolic self-destruction. It's a bleak reality, but we can climb out of it. Most people want an esoteric answer to our health woes. They want multiple studies and scientific conclusions, but that's a waste of time. The solution is simply increasing those woeful 205 calories to a more respectable number, as a percentage of total calories.

Based on discussions with my clients, by age 30 everyone is aware of some health issue he or she may have to grapple with. Many of them are fully aware it is due to what they eat and drink, but it is not too alarming. By age 40 it grabs their full attention, as they can feel its agitation and pain creeping into their bodies. Lo and behold, by age 50, it is a full-scale battle. They are usually forced to do something about it immediately. The doctor may give a bleak prognosis and suggest the "appropriate" medication to thwart any physical threats (e.g. heart attacks, strokes, dizziness, acute pain, irritable bowels, etcetera), but most of those battles could be averted or mitigated simply by changing what we put in our mouths for nutritive value, as well as pleasure. Again, that 8% of calories from fruits and veggies must be increased through frequent trips to the first aisle of the grocery store, the farmer's market or by any means where you can acquire fresh produce.

When you receive enlightening and practical knowledge, execute a disciplined game plan and maintain faith in what nature has provided, the healing process becomes easy and you start to feel younger. But, unfortunately, even with enlightenment and practical knowledge, many of us don't make positive food choices. Many will not adjust when they see the light, but only when they feel the heat of metabolic disaster. Therefore, before any disaster strikes, it all boils down to giving your body what it "truly" desires so it may function optimally; not falling prey to what your palate "capriciously" desires to get through any given moment.

Don't Diet, Eat with Style

To be healthy and happy we must implement a methodology to satisfy our true desires and keep life exciting by entertaining our caprices every now and then. It is impossible to be Goody Two-Shoes all the time, only eating what we know is best for us. We all have that dark side that says, "Eat that chocolate cake and ice-cream." The key is not to overindulge, which is the natural tendency. What makes REV so easy to implement is that it is not a diet that shuns the dark side of the psyche. Diets are short-term solutions that often backfire in the long term. REV is an eating style that could span the entirety of your life. It's geared toward producing a desired result based on understanding what food can and will do for you.

Your palate is not denied any type of food because it is "bad" for you, so there's no guilt involved. If you desire fried chicken, potato chips and ice cream—foods that could produce undesirable results—go for it and enjoy chewing. Just understand, without complaint, what doors you may be opening as a result. The objective of REV is to incorporate a greater percentage of fruits and vegetables into your eating style—that's it. If done in progressive stages, it will give you an enhanced understanding of the power of plant-based eating. Along with that enhanced understanding, you'll get some welcomed "desired" results. The beauty is that it takes minimal effort and it is stress free. Honestly, it's too easy.

As a compromise there will be foods not recommended for consumption, but not banned. To the detriment of many, junk food, comfort food, highly processed food, meat and dairy are commonplace in American culture. Since so many of us purportedly derive pleasure from those foods, it is unreasonable to suggest we wipe them off the face of the earth. Currently they maintain an unshakeable position in our social fabric. Only time will tell if those foods will continue to hold us hostage and drive metabolic syndrome.

Is There an Ideal Ratio?

REV is not intended to be conversion to a whole food plant-based eating style (although, metabolically speaking, whole food plant-based eating is the best way to go). It progresses you toward your ideal ratio of raw fruits

> *I believe that eating simple food in a healthy body with a clean conscience is more pleasurable, and infinitely more satisfying, than eating decadent food that makes you and your world ill. – John Robbins*

and veggies, cooked fruits and veggies, meats, dairy and processed food consumption by becoming a First Aisler. There is no agreed upon rule, nor is there a nutritional study which pins down the "ideal" ratio of how one should eat. There are too many cultures around the world that violate certain rules and seem to thrive (i.e., the French Paradox).

This book is based on the lifestyle and observations of yours truly, a personal trainer at a gym, observing what has worked for many. I would say, without a doubt, that 100% of my clients have benefited from incorporating more fruits and veggies into their eating styles. I've had many who have fought me for years on doing so, but when they do embrace the concept, nothing but good things start to happen, especially in the areas of weight loss and enhanced energy. With that in mind, the most important thing I could ever say about what food to eat is to let your level of energy determine what is best for you (*see Appendix B – The Age of the Resultatarian*). We all want that perfect formula based on rigorous scientific studies, but that does not seem to be working out too well for the masses. It is time to stop relying on expert opinions and diagnoses that may not have your best interest at heart. Your body responds to stimuli and activity. If you listen to it closely, you will get all the answers you need to live a higher quality life.

Please understand that we certainly do need experts in our lives, as they are vital to our existence. However, they should be consulted after we've done our due diligence at the food table. It makes no sense to go to a health professional if you're putting garbage in your body. All you will get are prescriptions and recommendations to help you manage the garbage with its related health consequences. Even the Judeo-Christian tradition begins with the concept of plant-based eating. In Genesis 1:29, God said in the Garden of Eden, "I give you every seed-bearing plant on the face of the whole earth and every tree that has fruit with seed in it. They will be yours for food." If we follow that directive first, then seek professional help when we have health challenges, our doctors, dieticians and other professionals will be much more effective. Just keep in mind that everything we need for supreme energy and radiance grows in a garden.

How to Get the Job Done?

REV is here to help us discover the "right direction" by becoming more harmonious with nature. It is a starter kit to transition to a first aisle eating style. There are not many references to studies and medical trials, nor is there a lot of science to support what is written, but there are references to common sense. That said, there would be heavy criticism on that point, but I must follow the path that produces the best results that I have seen, short term and long term. Therefore, don't expect esoteric revelations or discovery of nutritional secrets. They do not exist. Personally, I've never heard advice better than "an apple a day keeps the doctor away". If you like, substitute "an apple" with any fruit or vegetable you fancy and the advice is still effective.

REV is a 6-step process. Each step I suggest you engage in for two to three weeks. If you need more time, take it. You'll get information regarding why you are asked to take each step, some statistics to accentuate certain points, as well as some client anecdotes and personal reflections. If you follow each step, in three months you'll be a new and improved person. I'd bet my last nickel that 90% of your health issues will be mitigated, with some being completely eradicated. Also, you do not have to take every step to benefit from REV. If you stop at step three or four, you'll be way ahead of the game. Take your time and enjoy the ride.

My journey into plant-based eating took three years, back in the 1980s. I had no idea I was moving in that direction, but as I refrained from animal products more and more, I felt stronger. There was no plan because I didn't even know what "veganism" was. However, in today's time, there are more resources for those interested in plant-based eating. Also, I started at 25 years of age as a young man. You may be older with metabolic issues. That said, it's best to get started right away and accelerate the process.

Don't Get Offended

As aforementioned, you're not precluded from eating any type of food. After thousands of conversations with clients I've learned that if I tell someone to give up something, he or she may miss the whole point of the process. I've also learned that food and drink are highly emotional subjects and integral parts of cultures and societies around the world. They produce far more pleasure than sex and drugs for most people; they are sacred for others. Many people are "married" to certain types of food and only death will sever them from it, so they take offense when asked to sacrifice it for the greater good.

Quite some time ago, I had a friend who suffered from gout. He knew which foods would trigger intense pain—namely spare ribs. I'd drive by the local rib shack and far too many times he'd be in line waiting to get his fix. I begged him to stop, but at that time he said he was willing to pay the price and suffer the consequences. Eventually he did stop, but only after much irreversible damage was done. It was very unfortunate, so I ask that you be reasonable. Sometimes you must be willing to sacrifice that which you love the most. Treating your body like a temple—not like a woodshed—is your best option.

> *I've found that if I tell somebody "Eat this and don't do that," it's not only not helpful, it's counterproductive because even more than being healthy, we want to feel free and in control, and as soon as somebody tells us to do something, there's a tendency to do just the opposite. -- Dean Ornish, MD*

Once I asked a client to give up coffee for a few weeks. She was suffering from migraines and I suspected caffeine was the culprit. She fought me tooth and nail to defend the "virtues" of coffee and caffeine. Every morning the great joy of her life was that she and her husband would stroll to Starbucks and enjoy a cup of coffee to get revved up and start their day. That morning ritual was sacred to her, but I felt obligated to let her know of the potential cause and cure for her migraines. To my dismay, she took my advice as a personal attack against her intelligence and she never made the sacrifice. Sad to say she continues to struggle.

Another time I asked a client to give up dairy products for her entire family because her kids were frequently sick and missed many days from school. After studying the effects of dairy, I'm convinced it's an extremely dangerous product, especially for children. My suggestion was soy, rice, hemp or almond milk as an alternative—anything but cow's milk. That client took it as a personal attack against her parenting skills, although I never said she was a bad mom. Thereafter, she refused to listen to anything I had to say regarding food choices, although her children suffered from myriad allergies, digestive issues and skin allergies, possibly due to dairy consumption. Apparently, the doctors she consulted didn't seem to have a clue. Unfortunately, her children's pain continued.

Because of those incidents, and many others, I tread lightly when sharing information or giving advice. I rarely ask clients to sacrifice any food or drink, unless they want an immediate catapult into plant-based eating. When feasible, I prefer that they incorporate a food or drink that hopefully squeezes out what I would otherwise ask to be sacrificed for the greater good. My responsibility is to give the best advice I'm aware of, not to attack anyone. Therefore, REV is full of suggestions, not directives. Educating yourself is of prime importance. Again, I stress that nothing is restricted from the food table, just beware of the consequences of your food choices, based primarily on how your body responds. If you back that up with your own research, health and youth is yours for the taking. The average American is digging his own grave with a spoon, fork and knife; but you can also fortify your temple with those same utensils.

> *We should all be eating fruits and vegetables as if our lives depend on it, because they do. – Michael Greger, MD*

Step 1 – Water, Water Everywhere

Second to oxygen, water is our most important need. A human being can live approximately six days without it. When you do not have enough water your organs begin to shut down and those days are quite ugly. Yet, with as much water as we have access to in this country, most Americans are doing themselves a disservice by not taking advantage of it. We may think we are hydrated properly, but the stats are saying something different. According to MedicalDaily.com, 75% of Americans may suffer from chronic dehydration.[17] Water maintains the balance of body fluids, it energizes muscles, clears the skin, improves kidney function, neutralizes and dilutes the acidity of your blood, eases bowel movements and reduces caloric intake. Certainly we want variety to quench our thirst, but the quest for variety is the beginning of our unraveling. When you are amply hydrated your body functions much more efficiently and effectively. Therefore, your primary focus must be to get enough water into your body on a daily basis.

> *I believe that water is the only drink for a wise man.*
> *-- Henry David Thoreau*

Which Water is Best?

This is a tough question to answer because our water supply is not as pure as we may desire. Since the 2014 catastrophe of excessive lead in the Flint, Michigan water supply, everyone has become concerned about water quality and safety. We seem to have many choices of which water to consume.

1. *Drinking Water.* Called tap water and usually comes from a municipal source. It contains no added ingredients, except what is considered "safe" for human consumption, such as fluoride.

2. *Distilled Water.* A type of purified water that has gone through a filtration process to strip away contaminants and natural minerals.

3. *Purified Water.* Water that comes from any source, but has been purified through distillation, deionization, reverse osmosis or carbon filtration to remove harmful chemicals and/or beneficial minerals.

4. *Spring Water.* Water from an underground source that may or may not have been treated and purified. This is what we normally get in bottled water.

At this stage of REV there is no preference regarding which water to drink, provided it is not contaminated. In the ideal world we would all drink fresh spring water because it contains natural minerals that are beneficial to us. However, I would suggest distilled or purified just to be sure nothing dangerous is in the water.

Be careful of mineral enhanced water since many brands contain harmful chemicals. For instance, Dasani, Smart Water and Nestle's Pure Life contain chemicals such as magnesium sulfate, potassium chloride, calcium chloride, magnesium chloride, potassium bicarbonate, sodium bicarbonate, and magnesium sulfate.[18] All those ingredients are not necessary, they are just added for enhanced taste. The amounts are small enough to be considered safe by governmental agencies, but do they have a negative cumulative effect over the long term? There is no definitive answer to that question, but I would steer clear of mineral enhanced water.

How Much is Enough?

What is the perfect amount of water for maximum energy and performance? There is a conventional formula which says divide your body weight in half. The number you get should be the number of ounces of water you should drink. I weigh 195 pounds; therefore, I should drink 97.5 ounces of water each day. This may be a great way to calculate your water needs, but it does not consider your physical activity or lack thereof. For example, on a steamy day on the tennis court, I may drink a gallon in an hour or two, then more later during the day. The next day I may not exercise at all and I will only need a couple of quarts. In those scenarios there is a variance of 64 to 256 ounces, so the conventional formula does not work very well.

The urine color test is a much better indicator. You are properly hydrated when your urine is clear to a very light yellowish color. The deeper yellow it is the more water you need to start drinking. There are two things that will determine the color of your urine: how much water your body stores and how much it eliminates (sweat, exhalation, urination, bowel movements, etc.). Considering those two factors, the amount of water one needs each day may vary greatly.

Water Always Comes First

Make it your first task of the day to drink water. Wake up and drink a pint of water as soon as you get out of the bed. Do not put anything in your system until you have consumed water first.

Putting water into your digestive system before all else will do a couple of positive things for you. First, the more water you drink, the less likely it will be that you will drink anything acidic or harmful. I've had many clients who prefer coffee as their first beverage of the day. Many do not feel as though they can function without that early morning caffeine jolt. They are addicted to it, willfully admit it, and steadfastly refuse to discuss curtailing it, even the slightest bit.

Caffeine is Dangerous

Caffeine is a highly addictive drug. There are many who have tried to give it up, but suffered from complications similar to those who are detoxing from other recreational drugs. If you have ever experienced caffeine withdrawal symptoms it should be a clear indicator that there is a serious problem.

There was a time when I consumed coffee like it was going out of style, especially when I worked the graveyard shift in a computer lab. Before each shift I would drink two huge Dunkin Donuts coffees, loaded with sugar and milk, and I'd throw in two chocolate chip cookies for an extra sugar boost. Then, mid-shift, I'd have another big coffee. Coffee, sugar and milk are too much of an acid overload for the human body to handle over an extended period of time.

According to *CaffeineInformer.com* there are *18 Harmful Effects of Caffeine*[19] *(please view the website for references)*

20 Harmful Effects of Caffeine

1. More than 4 cups of coffee linked to early death.
2. Caffeine consumption may raise blood pressure.
3. Increased risk of heart attack among young adults.
4. Caffeine linked to gout attacks.
5. Breast tissue cysts in women.
6. Caffeine could cause incontinence.
7. Caffeine may cause insomnia.
8. Caffeine can cause indigestion.
9. Caffeine can cause headaches.
10. Caffeine could reduce fertility in women.
11. Caffeine may not be healthy for type 2 diabetics.
12. Caffeine and miscarriage risk.
13. Caffeine overdose.
14. Caffeine allergies.
15. Caffeine causes more forceful heart contractions.
16. Worse Menopause Symptoms.
17. Caffeine consumption can lead to increased anxiety, depression and the need for anxiety medication.
18. Caffeine increases the amount of sugary beverages consumed by people.
19. Caffeine inhibits collagen production in skin.
20. Caffeine interferes with ossification and could also lead to greater risk of bone loss.

Those 20 reasons are pretty bleak. During my days as a habitual coffee drinker, it never crossed my mind that coffee might be harmful. But, if that's not enough to prompt you to take action, here's a little more to think about: *The Top 15 Caffeine Withdrawal Symptoms* are[20]:

Top 15 Caffeine Withdrawal Symptoms

1. Headache
2. Sleepiness
3. Irritability
4. Lethargy
5. Constipation
6. Depression
7. Muscle Pain, Stiffness, Cramping
8. Lack of Concentration
9. Flu-like symptoms
10. Insomnia
11. Nausea and Vomiting
12. Anxiety
13. Brain Fog
14. Dizziness
15. Heart Rhythm Abnormalities

Who wants to deal with any of those withdrawal symptoms? Unfortunately, I know quite a few people who would battle through many of them. They've experienced them in the past and they're struck with fear to experience them again, so they continue to consume caffeine. They get their energy boost and grind through the day. To many those consequences may not seem that bad because we all know older people who drink coffee daily and appear to be just fine. The real question is how much energy do you want during the advanced stages of your life? As mild as caffeine may seem and as pleasurable as it may be, any drug addiction will only detract from your energy resources. You may be able to get away with it for the moment, but it always catches up with you.

To be fair, there are those who extoll the virtues of green tea. Many will argue that the caffeine in green tea improves brain functioning and physical performance. In addition, there are claims that it has many other therapeutic qualities, such as preventing Alzheimer's Disease, Parkinson's Disease, cancer and heart disease. Therefore, I encourage you to investigate it further, keeping in mind that caffeine is a drug. Like any other drug, if abused, it could be the beginning of your unraveling.

Is Milk as Pure White as It Seems?

Many younger people have been conditioned to start the day off with a little protein and calcium jolt from cow's milk. However, this can be disruptive to the digestive system and even dangerous for certain segments of the population. Many would argue that cow's milk increases the acidity of your blood and introduces harmful hormones and proteins into your system. There has been serious debate on this subject and a consensus has yet to be achieved.

The real question is, should humans consume the milk of another species? The dairy industry argues we need it to build strong bones, and they have the coolest milk mustache ads to accentuate the point. But, biologically speaking, cow's milk is designed to double the size of a newborn calf in 45 to 50 days. Humans do not grow that fast. It takes a newborn human child six months to double in size. Since cows grow much more rapidly, cow's milk contains almost three times the amount of protein than human breast milk. Biologically, we are not designed to handle that much protein, and this could eventually lead to myriad of complications. Yet, the National Dairy Council insists that we must get certain nutrients from milk (calcium, potassium, vitamin D) or risk suffering the consequences of stroke, hypertension, colon cancer or osteoporosis.[21] It is extremely confusing.

The irony is that there are many ethnic groups worldwide that have high percentages of lactose intolerance, some as high as 90%.[22] This point is particularly disturbing because many children in our public school systems are fed milk and cheese as part of their government sponsored food programs. Considering the dairy industry is highly subsidized by the government, it appears that someone must pay the price, and our kids are first in line. They are totally oblivious to the potential dangers they face, and so are most adults. Nevertheless, it is our duty to inform them of the risks. Here are the *11 Reasons to Stop Drinking Cow's Milk* from PETA.org. [23]

> ## *11 Reasons to Stop Drinking Cow's Milk (PETA.org)*
>
> *1. Broken bones*
> *2. Prostate cancer*
> *3. Lactose intolerance*
> *4. Acne*
> *5. Cholesterol*
> *6. Ovarian cancer*
> *7. Milk allergies*
> *8. Antibiotics*
> *9. Saturated fat*
> *10. Weight gain*
> *11. Bone loss*

Milk is the best option for a newborn, when it is human breast milk. Consuming animal milk, for the sake of more protein and calcium, is definitely not the best way to go in the long run.

Fruit Juice is Too Sweet

Another drink that we tend to view as "healthy" is fruit juice. Drinking natural fruit juices can be detrimental to your health. When they are consumed, we ingest a much more concentrated amount of sugar than our bodies are designed to handle. That sugar can then be packed away as fat. Eight ounces of orange juice contains 21 grams of sugar and 110 calories, while an average sized orange contains only 7 grams of sugar and 40 calories. However, most people drink more than eight ounces of juice. The smallest size in most convenience stores is a pint (16 ounces) that still may not be enough to satisfy an energetic kid or active adult. Personally, I can easily drink a quart at a time. However, eating a whole orange could be more satisfying than a pint of orange juice, with a sixth of the calories. The orange is a powerful fruit, full of antioxidants, phytonutrients and fiber. It is better to eat an orange than to drink its juice.

Soda isn't the Answer

Sugary soft drinks are even worse than natural fruit juices because highly concentrated sugar is added. There are more than 60 names for added sugar, including corn syrup, dextrose, evaporated cane juice, fruit juice concentrates, high-fructose corn syrup, diglycerides, disaccharides, sorghum, xylitol and zylose. When reading "nutrition facts" labels on soft drinks and other processed drinks, it is easy to be seduced into believing there is not a potent amount of sugar in the product. Those sugars provide nothing but empty calories. For instance, a 12-ounce can of soda contains approximately 8 teaspoons of added sugar with no other nutritive benefits (unless you consider the 50 milligrams of added sodium a benefit).[24] They provide no fiber, vitamins or minerals and without those nutrients, there is nothing left but a catalyst for metabolic disaster.

By the way, the added sugar daily consumption recommendation of the USDA is no more than 6 teaspoons for an adult woman. Obviously, one can of soda is far beyond that and could be considered dangerous for your health.

Artificial Sweeteners

The FDA has approved five artificial sweeteners: saccharin, acesulfame, aspartame, neotame and sucralose. It has also approved one natural, low-calorie sweetener, stevia. For me, artificial sweeteners are a gray area. I cannot say they are good or bad in my experience because I have never used them. One knock against them is that people may over-consume non-nutritious foods that contain them. Because they are consuming fewer calories, they feel they can get away with it. Also, another concern is that the Multi-Ethnic Study of Atherosclerosis by the American Diabetes Association reported that artificial sweeteners in diet soda might contribute to a rise in metabolic syndrome.[25] Since they are artificial and have side effects, in general I would suggest avoiding them. Aspartame (sold under brand names "NutraSweet" and "Equal") is known to be toxic because it forms methanol when heated, which then converts into formaldehyde in the body.[26] In small quantities this may not be harmful, but since Americans consume so much processed food we should all be on guard. Aspartame is found in more than 6,000 products worldwide and it is the most consumed artificial sweetener in the U.S.A. Because it is marketed as safer and healthier than sugar, we tend to believe that products that contain it (especially diet sodas) are a safe alternative, but there is much evidence to refute those claims. Common symptoms of Aspartame consumption are headaches and migraines, as well as weight gain.[27]

Stevia is a natural sweetener derived from a plant native to Brazil and Paraguay. It is approximately 200 times sweeter than sugar. It has been used for over 1,500 years as a sweetener and for treatment for burns, stomach problems, colic and even for contraception. There does not appear to be serious side effects of stevia; therefore, I would recommend it over artificial sweeteners. However, I would suggest using it cautiously, if at all.

Alcohol is Poison

Is there any debate about the dangers of alcoholic beverages? Many people thoroughly enjoy a glass of wine or a few sips of scotch, and they should be allowed to do so. Admittedly I have enjoyed my fair share. Yet, you must recognize that alcohol is poisonous to your system. Short term, it distorts your brain processes, ranging from relaxing your inhibitions to becoming flat drunk. Long term it can disrupt your liver functioning, causing myriad metabolic problems. In his YouTube video, "Sugar: The Bitter Truth", Robert Lustig, M.D. informs his audience that excessive, long term alcohol consumption has been linked to many of the same metabolic diseases as excessive, long term fructose consumption.[28] Those diseases include hypertension, myocardial infarction, dyslipidemia, pancreatitis, obesity, hepatic dysfunction and addiction.

We can all agree it's unlikely that alcohol consumption around the world will ever end; therefore, it must be regulated by the government due to the serious public consequences such as public drunkenness, driving while intoxicated, etcetera. However, it is highly unlikely that the chronic effects will ever be regulated; therefore, we must be disciplined regarding its consumption. Enjoy it as a treat, but limit it.

Water: The Best Thing for Weight Loss

Overall, our population is in the worst shape it's ever been. Children are in terrible shape. We have absolutely unprecedented numbers of obese and overweight children - one in three now. A generation ago it was something like one in ten. – Neal Barnard, MD

One of the great benefits of drinking water when you first arise is that it diminishes your hunger for food that is high in preservatives, fat, sugar and salt. Donuts, muffins, cereals, pancakes, waffles and syrup are very harmful in that they pack on the pounds. Two-thirds of Americans are overweight and half of those are obese. There is even an epidemic of childhood obesity that we must consider. That said, anything that we can do to decrease the amount of calorically dense food we consume is highly advisable; and drinking more water is the most innocuous way to do this. According to the National Institutes of Health "Water consumption acutely reduces meal energy intake (EI) among middle-aged and older adults…Thus, when combined with a hypocaloric diet, consuming 500 ml of water prior to each main meal leads to greater weight loss than a hypocaloric diet alone in middle-aged and older adults."[29]

CALL TO ACTION

Objective: ***Drink water until your urine is clear.***

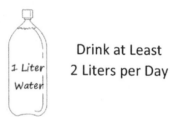

Drink at Least
2 Liters per Day

How do we seamlessly integrate more water into our lifestyles? First start the day off by drinking at least a pint of water. Finish the pint before drinking or eating anything else. Enjoy your coffee, tea, hot chocolate or orange juice, but after drinking your allotment of water.

For those who are zealous about staying young, as I am, you must first drink at least a quart of water before imbibing or eating anything. As soon as I wake up I chug down a pint. If you keep a container of water right by your bedside, this will also help with the process. Next, I get dressed for work and chug down another pint. When you do so you will immediately feel full and your hunger decreases.

Second, always have water near you. When possible carry a bottle of it with you all day. If you have the desire for something acidic or sugary, enjoy a few sips of water first. It's guaranteed you'll drink less of what you know can cause you harm. You'll also start breaking any sugar addictions you may have.

Third, keep water in your car. If you drive a lot, oftentimes you may pull over for something to munch on or drink during your trip. As you walk into a convenience store you may be seduced by the smell of coffee and the colorful soft drink bottles, but you must not succumb so easily. Knowing you have your safety bottle of water in the car will help you to resist the charm and guile of the advertisers. If you do break down and buy something loaded with sugar or caffeine, you won't fall too far off track. (By the way, flavored water is not recommended because most brands contain refined sugars, food coloring and other chemicals.)

For many, drinking a lot of water within three to four hours of going to bed is not the best idea. If you drink too much, then your sleep may be interrupted to make a few too many trips to the commode. There may also be interrupted sleep if you eat lots of high water content food, which are many fruits and vegetables. Personally, I have a water cut-off and I do not drink much after 6pm, unless I'm exercising during the evening. It is great to be aggressive with hydrating, but be reasonable. A good night's sleep is vital to your health!

As you drink more and more water, notice how you feel. According to my clients, they feel more energetic and more restful during the evening. Having fewer toxic chemicals in your body won't put as much of a drain on your metabolic processes. Drink often, drink well and stay young!

If there is magic on this planet, it is contained in water.

Loran Isley

Step 2 – Enjoy Your Dessert

Beyond a shadow of a doubt, fruit is the turning point of REV. Eating fruit will unlock your potential and put you on the fast track to health and happiness! Unfortunately, in the greatest country in the world, fruit consumption is not given its due respect. It does not get many food advertisements because it's not considered comfort food. Supposedly it's not sweet enough, so cupcakes and donuts are more marketable. Let's face it: it's not deemed something "fun" to eat. As we're constantly bombarded with ads for mass-produced and chemically induced foods, the best food is right at our fingertips and we don't even realize it.

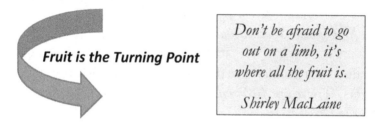

Fruit is the Turning Point

Don't be afraid to go out on a limb, it's where all the fruit is.

Shirley MacLaine

Are You a Sugar Addict?

One day a client told me her favorite snack is Fat-Free Twizzlers. We had a heated discussion about it when another lady jumped in and said, "It says fat-free on the label, it's healthy!" I asked, "What about the processed sugar in it?" Her response, "Uhh…"

The beauty of fruit is that it contains the magic ingredient that drives us wild: sugar! We must face the fact that Americans are sugar addicts. We live it; we breathe it.

However, the problem is that the average American is having a love affair with processed and refined sugars. It's hard to get away from it when it's in 74% of processed foods![30] By law, as of 2017, food manufacturers are required to list the total amount of sugar in their products, but they are not required to list how much is "added" sugar. Because of this, it should be obvious that the amount of sugar you're ingesting is way beyond the normal amounts intended by nature.

> *One of the leading causes of obesity is the misbelief that, when it comes to juice, "100%" means sugar-free.*
> *— Mokokoma Mokhonoana*

The table sugar and high fructose corn syrup that we love so dearly is highly addictive. I have plenty of clients who are addicted to it and don't even realize it. Frankly, it's a drug like cocaine, just milder on the body and without the acute effects. There are *10 Similarities Between Sugar, Junk Food and Abusive Drugs.*[31]

1. Studies have shown that sugar and junk foods flood the reward system in the brain with dopamine, stimulating the same areas as drugs of abuse like cocaine.
2. Cravings are a common symptom when it comes to both junk foods and addictive drugs, and have very little to do with actual hunger.
3. Scientists have used functional MRI (fMRI) scanners to show that the same brain regions are

activated in response to cues and cravings for both junk foods and drugs.

4. When the brain's reward system is repeatedly over-stimulated, it responds by reducing its number of receptors. This leads to tolerance, one of the hallmarks of addiction.

5. Binge eating is a common symptom of food addiction. It is caused by increasing tolerance, making the brain need a larger dose than before to reach the same effect.

6. Studies have shown that addicted rats can switch between sugar, amphetamine and cocaine. This is called "cross-sensitization" and is one feature of addictive substances.

7. Drugs that are used to fight addictions such as smoking, alcoholism and heroin-addiction, are also effective for weight loss. This indicates that food affects the brain in similar ways as these drugs of abuse.

8. There is plenty of evidence in rats that abstaining from sugar and junk food can lead to clear withdrawal symptoms.

9. It is common knowledge that junk foods are harmful, but many people are still unable to control their consumption.

10. Food addiction symptoms satisfy the official medical criteria for addiction.

Robert H. Lustig, M.D., Professor of Pediatrics at the University of California, San Francisco, believes excessive fructose consumption is the driving force behind metabolic syndrome in America.[32] In the early 1900s the average fructose consumption in America was about 15 grams per person, per day. In 1997, the average fructose consumption for adolescents 12 to 18 years of age was about 73 grams per person per day.[33] Many would agree that an increase of almost 500% is certainly not in your best interest. Not to mention the number keeps rising.

> *Sweeteners, which can be up to 300 times sweeter than natural sugar, are known to increase appetite and result in overeating. Be on the lookout for artificial sweeteners, and when possible, steer clear of them. – Mehmet Oz, MD*

Table sugar is approximately 50% glucose and 50% fructose. High fructose corn syrup is slightly different, approximately 55% fructose and 45% glucose. When consuming those mixtures of processed sugar, the body immediately uses glucose, but fructose metabolizes differently. It is metabolized mainly by the liver, which becomes overloaded with the excessive quantities of fructose that the average American consumes. According to Dr. Lusting, after a certain period of abuse, one can develop non-alcoholic fatty liver disease (NAFLD) and as we know, metabolic syndrome is on the loose. Essentially fructose is metabolized as poisons are and it is extremely dangerous over the course of a lifetime. It insidiously causes weight gain by "not" triggering satiety signals to the brain. Essentially your brain doesn't know you're satiated after eating many sugary products, so you continue to eat. What follows are the diseases associated with metabolic syndrome, including diabetes and obesity. Consequently, diabetes and obesity rates in America and the world are escalating out of control. For instance, in 1980 approximately 108 million people worldwide had diabetes. That number has risen about 400% to 422 million in 2014. The World Health Organization estimates that number will double in the next 20 years if current trends continue.[34]

The Raw Power of Fruit

Of course, you might be wondering how can fruit help since it contains sugar? When I talk to people at the gym and they say, "I don't eat fruit because it has too much sugar in it," it makes me want to cry. Cutting out fruit is ridiculous! The fact is anywhere in nature where we are given sugar in its natural state, we're also given fiber to protect us. Fiber is the great neutralizer which slows down the absorption rate of sugar. Since there is less sugar and insulin in your bloodstream at a given moment, less sugar is stored away as fat and more is burned for energy. Also, fiber fills you up and satiates you without adding calories. It is the magic ingredient for weight control and fruit has an abundance of it. If you truly want to lose weight, do not eat anything without natural fiber in it. It works like a charm.

Aside from fiber, fruit contains valuable vitamins, minerals and phytonutrients that are stripped away during food processing. Those vitamins, minerals and phytonutrients work better together, in their natural state, compared to working in isolation when they are mass-produced. When processed food is "fortified" some of those vitamins and minerals are put back in the processed food. It certainly does not make the processed food any stronger. In fact, it may not enhance the potency or value of the food at all. Additionally, harmful chemicals may be used during the extraction and fortification processes, so do not be deluded and fall into the trap of eating "fortified" foods believing that you are getting something powerful from them.

Is Sugar Really a Problem?

> *Sugar gave rise to the slave trade; now sugar has enslaved us. — Jeff O'Connell*

The reason that fruit is the turning point in REV is because we must turn our backs on sugar addiction once and for all. Sugar has been demonized over the last thirty years as we have ventured into the "low-carb" era with popular diets. As America has become more and more fat, most are clinging to the notion that low-carb and high protein is the way to go. We have latched onto ketogenic diets (e.g., the Atkin's Diet, South Beach Diet) as if they are the messiahs for our obesity woes. But, we must embrace sugar for what it really is: a carbohydrate that our bodies must have which should be consumed from a "natural source." Fruit is the perfect natural source.

Human beings are primates and as such we are blessed with the ability to taste sweetness in food where other animals cannot. As a matter of fact, the "sweet pleasure" sensation is so powerful it can mask the other tastes. For instance, when food manufacturers offer their products to the marketplace that are salty, sour or bitter, adding a little sugar can make them more palatable. Items like sweet and sour pork, sugary chocolate bars and salty pretzels would waste away on the shelves if their added sugars were removed.

America was on a low-fat craze back in the 1970s and 80s, as fat had been demonized as the cause for our heart disease and obesity woes. Fat was then removed from many processed foods, but those foods lost their flavor along with the fat. Obviously, that created a serious problem for the food manufacturers, as sales would plummet. But, here comes sugar to save the day! When it is added to fat-free, tasteless food, it gives it that zest for enhanced palatability. Order is then restored; and the product flies off the shelf. Ironically, the calories subtracted by taking the fat out are packed back in by increasing the sugar content. As a result, obesity rates have continued to climb and we are nowhere near the end of the ascent. Based on a study reported by the National Institute of Health in 2009-10, "Linear time trend forecasts suggest that by 2030, 51% of the population will be obese. The model estimates a much lower obesity prevalence of 42% and severe obesity prevalence of 11%. If obesity were to remain at 2010 levels, the combined savings in

> *Eating crappy food isn't a reward— it's a punishment.*
> *– Drew Carey*

medical expenditures over the next 2 decades would be $549.5 billion."[35]

Lastly, sugar makes you age faster. According to *14 Foods That Make You Look Older,* when you ingest excessive amounts of sugar, your body cannot handle it. The sugar molecules bind with proteins in your body and cause glycation, which destroys your cells. When sugar combines with collagen it deteriorates your skin, making you look older.[36]

One of my weaknesses is chocolate chip scones from Whole Foods. There were periods where I would eat one or two a day for a month. Then I would kick the habit, but jump right back into the abyss a couple of months later. Another issue was eating cake and donuts at vegan restaurants in Manhattan. Whether cake is vegan or not, it is still loaded with processed sugars. Whenever I went overboard with scones and cake, my skin would pay the price as I would see bumps pop up on my face a day or so later. I never thought of myself as eating too much or being a sugar addict, but just a little bit was enough to throw me off my game. I can only imagine what the sugar was doing to my internal organs and metabolism. If you're serious about staying young, processed sugar must be cut to a bare minimum.

Processed sugar has a powerful position in American culture. Its prominence is rooted in finding the "bliss point" for food where it's most pleasing to us. Dr. Howard Moskowitz, affectionately nicknamed "Dr. Bliss," was a long-time food industry consultant. He and others in the food industry were charged with finding the exact combinations of sugar, fat and salt which bring the most pleasure to human beings, "And it's Howard who coined the expression 'bliss point' to

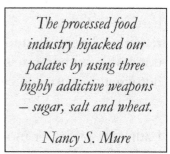

The processed food industry hijacked our palates by using three highly addictive weapons – sugar, salt and wheat.

Nancy S. Mure

capture that perfect amount of sweetness that would send us over the moon."[37] It is no mistake that sugar is added to 74% of processed food. It was a brilliant design to get people to buy more and eat more and it continues to work without fail. But beware! It is a grave we're digging with forks, spoons and knives almost every time we enjoy those morsels of processed food.

CALL TO ACTION

Objective: ***Eat at least 6 pieces of fruit per day!***

In this step of REV your mission is to dig yourself out of that sugar pit you may be in by eating at least six pieces of fruit throughout your day. It does not matter when, it does not matter where, just eat it. The objective is for fruit to be what you consume when you habitually reach for something sugary and processed. By allowing it to become your "go to" food, it can help break your processed sugar addiction. The cravings that you have for super sweet, sugar-laden processed food will diminish by replacing it with something naturally sweet, unprocessed and super healthy. The beauty of it is that you don't have to work hard to achieve the six piece per day objective, it just requires discipline and time. You may go through noticeable withdrawal symptoms from processed sugar, but when you are addicted to any substance, that is to be expected.

Eating six pieces or more of fruit per day gets you in the habit of experiencing sugar in its natural state. Most eating is habitual and many of us eat for recreation when we are not even hungry. Sugar in its natural form, in fruits and other plants, is not the demon we should be battling. To the contrary, it is an angel we must embrace. Processed sugar is the predator we must annihilate. Think for a moment: How many times have you thought that Justin ate too many bananas or Jennifer ate too many apples, it is no wonder they're overweight. Probably never! But, we can all name droves of people who are overweight from eating too many Krispy Kreme Donuts, French fries, potato chips and other sugar-infused processed foods. Sometimes, we must look at the obvious to understand the seemingly complex. Americans are habitually conditioned to eat processed foods and we must recondition ourselves to eat fruit.

Reason number two for eating six pieces of fruit per day, is that you will probably get sick and tired of eating it before it makes you sick and tired. As far as I know, there is no upper limit of fruit consumption that is hazardous to your health; however, we are assuming raw fruit, in its natural state, will be consumed. No candied apples, chocolate covered strawberries, fruit smoothies with honey or any type of dried fruits. And yes, six pieces of fruit sounds like a lot—especially when most people eat none—but it certainly won't devastate you like eating the same volume of cake and ice cream will. As a matter of fact, Dr. Michael Greger reports that fruit is, "beneficial in almost any amount" based on a Harvard Health Letter article, "Rethinking Fructose in Your Diet" in July of 2013.[38]

Six pieces of fruit is a drop in the bucket calorie-wise compared to what the average American is consuming in processed sugar. For instance, six oranges are approximately 250 calories; six bananas are approximately 540 calories. If you eat just one Caramel Crunch Krispy Kreme donut, you will consume 390 calories, and there are few people who only eat just one. Additionally, you are getting minimal nutritive value from the donut, if any, but you will be getting loads of antioxidants, minerals, phytochemicals and fiber from the fruit. Sounds like a no-brainer. Simply put, fruit is not the bad guy.

What types of fruit should you eat? It is totally your choice. At this second stage of REV you are still transitioning; therefore, the objective is to get fruit in your system. You do not need to be sidetracked regarding which fruit is better than another since they are all pretty good. If you have not been enjoying any fruit at all or even very little up to this point in your life, then whichever fruit tickles your fancy will provide more vitamins, minerals, and anti-oxidants than you would have ever bargained for.

When and where you eat your six pieces of fruit per day is a personal choice. As a suggestion, eating two pieces before breakfast, lunch and dinner is an extremely effective method. If you are hungry for breakfast and you eat fruit first, you will probably have less desire for cereal, bacon, eggs, grits or pancakes. It is a safe and effective way of quelling the desire to eat other foods that may pack on the calories and sap your energy.[39]

Once I had a client who was in love with pizza, but he knew it was weighing him down on the scale. At least five times a week he would make a late-night pit stop at the pizza parlor before going home. I told him do not stop eating the pizza; just eat one piece of fruit for every slice of pizza he intended to eat. That evening he ate three bananas, but he could only eat one slice of pizza. The next couple of nights he did the same thing. In less than a week he was feeling more energized and lighter than ever.

Many people prefer to make their fruit into a smoothie. This method is not recommended because people tend to over-consume by using too many pieces of fruit at one time. For instance, eating two bananas fills me up, but I will throw four and some strawberries into a smoothie. Then most people toss in other ingredients, such as sweeteners and protein powders. This may improve the taste of your fruit smoothie, but it could be hazardous to your health over the long run (this will be covered in a later chapter). It is always best to eat your fruit instead of juicing or blending it, so juice it and blend it sparingly.

Consuming more fruit (at least 6 pieces a day) is the turning point of your journey toward a first aisle eating style. It is time to take advantage of what is best for you and what tastes best. It will keep you younger than ever. That's a guarantee!

Warning: too much fruit causes HEALTH!

Step 3 – Break Your Fast

Everything you put in your mouth and chew on is important, but it is critical that your first meal of the day builds positive momentum. Breakfast can set the sail for an energy filled morning, without the use of pick-me-up drugs. As you may have noticed, most people are sailing in the wrong direction. They are ships lost at sea with their only hope being caffeine and energy drinks.

Most of us wake up hungry and decide to break our fast with something highly processed. When I was a kid Pop Tarts were my favorite breakfast, with Eggo Waffles drowned in maple syrup a close second. Of course, I chewed on as much seared animal flesh as I could, sausage being my favorite. Back then I never thought about my poor little heart. I was eating recklessly and setting the stage for a host of metabolic diseases.

> *Eat breakfast like a king, lunch like a prince and dinner like a pauper. –*
> *Adelle Davis*

Let's Break Your Fast

To get on the right track your first meal of the day must focus on raw foods. Nothing processed, nothing cooked and, of course, as much water as you desire. The goal of step three of REV is to eat raw foods until lunchtime, at which time you may eat whatever you desire. If for some reason you cannot wait until lunch to have something processed or cooked, try to wait at least two hours after you have your fruit for breakfast.

We covered the virtues of fruit in the previous step, but there is a little more to add for step 3. The obvious question is what fruits to eat for breakfast? If you are allergic to a fruit, of course, it is out of the question. If you do not like the taste of a fruit, it is out of the question. REV is all about giving your taste buds exactly what they want. Every fruit you put in your mouth should be pure pleasure.

Personally, my fruit of choice depends on what activity I will be engaging in. If I am chilling out in the morning, my favorite fruits are cantaloupes or grapes. If I have a morning meeting where I must sit still for a time, I would not eat grapes because I will make too many trips to the restroom. If I am going to engage in strenuous activity, such as running or tennis, I prefer bananas and oranges.

In *The Best Pre-Workout Foods* in *Men's Health*, Dr. Louise Burke, head of Sports Nutrition at the Australian Institute of Sport, refers to bananas as "Nature's PowerBar". [40] I started eating bananas before and during

> *Some people who have been working out regularly for months or even years are still out of shape because the number of cheat days they have in a week exceeds six. — Mokokoma Mokhonoana*

workouts after watching tennis legend Michael Chang win the French Open in 1989. He had severe cramping issues, so he ate bananas during breaks between games. I have seen other professional tennis players do it also and I have not looked back. Your body needs electrolytes to fire on all cylinders, including potassium, calcium and sodium, along with other vitamins. Those minerals are critical for muscle contractions and endurance and bananas can fill that void.

Prior to and during exercise I do not advocate processed carbs, such as energy bars, unless there is no access to fresh fruit. They are normally laden with processed sugar, salt and other chemicals your body does not need. However, there are some exceptions. I've run a few half-marathons. Also, I ran an 8-mile Spartan race, up and down the side of a mountain, in dirt and mud (*I admit it was fun!*). Those strenuous activities may take two to five hours to complete and you will need lots of energy and endurance for the task. In extreme cases where I will have limited access to fresh food, I may put some energy bars in my fanny pack, just in case I get weak—sorry, but sometimes processed carbs may be your only choice. It is a better option than passing out trying to prove the point that raw foods are the only way to go. But, always remember, those processed foods are still dangerous when abused.

What Fruit is Best?

One fruit is not better than any other. Sure, in a laboratory you may be able to prove one has more vitamins and minerals than another, but that does not necessarily make it better. It depends on your body chemistry and metabolism. It also depends on what fruit you have access to. That said, there is no need to split hairs deciding which fruit is best.

However, just because you might be curious, *Time* recently published a list of *The 50 Healthiest Foods of All Time*.[41] Lo and behold, the top ten foods on the list are all fruits:

---

50 Healthiest Foods of All Time (Time Magazine)

1. Banana
2. Raspberry
3. Orange
4. Kiwi
5. Pomegranate
6. Blueberry
7. Grapefruit
8. Tangerine
9. Avocado
10. Tomato

Are You Nuts?

All you must do is walk into the first aisle of any supermarket and you can enjoy most of the fruits listed above. However, after eating fruit for breakfast many of my clients have complained that they still feel hungry. I then say, "Eat more fruit!" They then reply, "It doesn't fill me up!" It appears that many of us want a feeling of "fullness" that fruit may not provide for everyone. In keeping with a raw theme for breakfast, I would usually suggest eating a salad which is good at any time of day. The usual reaction is, "That's disgusting!" Most people I know consider salad for breakfast an apocalyptic event. Although salad is probably the best option, given that green, leafy veggies are the most nutrient dense foods we eat, most people want another option.

Raw nuts can be the answer to help get that "full" feeling, but this option can lead us into choppy waters. I have been an advocate of raw nuts, seeds and legumes for years, but it is possible they should be eaten in limited amounts. In fact, some in the health community believe that nuts should not be eaten at all, especially if you have heart disease. One of my heroes, Dr. Caldwell Essylstyn, a renowned physician regarding heart disease and author of *Prevent and Reverse Heart Disease*, believes in a diet, "Based on starches, vegetables, and fruits. No nuts, seeds, avocados, or other fatty plant foods are allowed. Emphasis is on eating very low-fat."[42] If you want to lose weight and cover all your bases, you may want to cut nuts out altogether.

There are, however, other opinions that encourage eating nuts. In 2013 an American Journal of Clinical Nutrition study concluded that, "Compared with control diets, diets enriched with nuts did not increase body weight, body mass index, or waist circumference in controlled clinical trials."[43] Given that there will always be conflicting opinions, as always, let your body tell you which way is best. I love nuts, especially raw cashews and pecans. From time to time I stop eating them because I tend to go overboard. However, I am not positive they contribute to any weight gain on my part.

Unfortunately, some people are allergic to nuts. According to FoodAllergy.org "Eight foods account for 90 percent of all reactions: milk, eggs, peanuts, tree nuts, soy, wheat, fish and shellfish. Even trace amounts of a food allergen can cause a reaction."[44] The Sydney Local Health District of Australia reported that peanuts cause the second most allergies in children, right behind eggs and before dairy products.[45] That said, be careful with nuts in your diet.

Which Nuts Are Best?

Like fruit, which nuts you prefer is an individual choice. It seems like everyone in the health community agrees that almonds are the best nutritionally, but no one really knows. We must simply develop the habit of consuming more raw nuts, so eat the ones you like the most. But, since you might be curious, here's a list of the most nutritious nuts. These nuts contain the

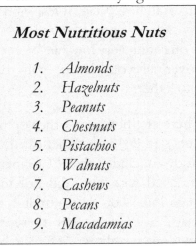

Most Nutritious Nuts

1. *Almonds*
2. *Hazelnuts*
3. *Peanuts*
4. *Chestnuts*
5. *Pistachios*
6. *Walnuts*
7. *Cashews*
8. *Pecans*
9. *Macadamias*

most protein, fiber, B-vitamins, calcium, minerals, and vitamin E with the least amount of saturated fat:[46]

Beware of "cooked" nuts. When nuts are roasted and laced with oil, salt, sugar, honey and only god knows what else, it can create problems for you. Some of the nutrients are lost and the chemical composition of them changes. And, by the way, "roasted" nuts are not really roasted. Anytime you see oil listed as an ingredient with "roasted nuts," the nuts are fried. "Dry roasted" nuts are not fried and do not contain any added oil.

How much should you eat? That depends on your appetite. REV does not limit the amount of raw food that you partake of, so simply listen to your body. If you eat too much you may feel sick or sluggish, therefore, start with a small handful and see how you feel. Personally, when I eat too much broccoli or spinach I feel uncomfortable, but when I eat too many cashews or pecans I feel sick. So, if you are a nut lover like me, it may be wise to put an upper limit on your nut consumption.

Fruit and Nuts Together?

Should you eat your fruit and nuts together? That is up to you. At the gym I am well known for eating bananas and nuts together. It all depends on whether you have positive digestive experiences doing so and what your ratio of fruits to nuts is. Your body will tell you the answer. Food combining is not something I have ever stressed in my lifestyle and is not a part of REV, although there may be great validity to it. I have heard arguments on both sides of the aisle on this topic. If you are a high-performance athlete, it is certainly a worthy topic to investigate. It may provide the winning edge you need.

Many people feel they need more protein, beyond what they get from fruits and veggies, to get that feeling of fullness. Raw nuts and seeds do provide a natural source of protein. Per ounce you will get about 4 to 6 grams of protein, along with other minerals, such as magnesium and calcium. The problem you will hear about nuts is that they are fattening. Yes, nuts contain a higher percentage of fats than most foods, but when your diet is filled with lots of raw fruits and vegetables, the fat in nuts would probably cause you little to no harm, provided you do not go overboard.

Starchy Veggies for Breakfast?

In addition to the fruit you consume for breakfast, cooked starchy veggies could be added when fruit is not filling enough. As great as raw fruits and veggies may be, many people still believe cooked food is just as good, if not superior. REV philosophy is in total agreement that cooked vegetables and grains have an important role in our metabolic vitality. Therefore, in addition to the fruit you consume for breakfast, cooked, starchy veggies could be added if you feel that fruit is not enough; but give fruit a chance!

Another of my heroes, John McDougall, MD, is the author of "The Starch Solution". For decades he has treated patients and educated the public on the virtues of a starch-based diet. Dr. McDougall believes, "The story is the same all over the world. Whether rice in Asia, potatoes in South America, corn in Central America, wheat in Europe, or beans, millet, sweet potatoes, and barley around the globe, starch has been at the center of food and nutrition throughout human history."[47]

For me, the best starchy veggies for energy are baked potatoes or sweet potatoes. We all know that potatoes have been vilified over the years and many people believe they are driving the obesity epidemic. That may be true if all you are eating are French fries and potato chips. However, it is completely unfair and nutritionally ridiculous to blame the potato. Potatoes provide a lot of energy without packing on the pounds. The problems arise when they are drenched in oil, fried, loaded with butter and dressed up with cheese. It is not the potato doing the damage, it is how it is prepared. French fries and potato chips are amongst the most physically devastating foods we eat, but a baked sweet potato, with nothing added to it, is heavenly. It is filling and only 90 calories. After eating a couple of those in the morning, you will get plenty of energy and you will feel satiated.

Years ago I would bathe my baked potatoes in olive oil, but I have since stopped that practice after learning about the harmful effects of oils. According to Joel Fuhrman, MD, "Ounce for ounce, olive oil is one of the most fattening, calorically dense foods on the planet; it packs even more calories per pound than butter (butter: 3,200 calories; olive oil: 4,020). The bottom line is that oil will add fat to our already plump waistlines, heightening the risk of disease, including diabetes and heart attacks."[48] Now I make my own oil free dressings. Sweet potatoes I can eat without adding anything to them. For those with limited time in the morning, all you must do is bake a batch of potatoes during the evening when you have a free hour. Store them in the fridge for later use and warm them up in the morning. I often chop a little onion and bell peppers and add that to them for additional flavor, then oil free dressing. From potatoes you get long lasting satiation that could last an entire morning. Dr. McDougall goes on to say, "Starches aren't just good for you, they're also satisfying. The abundant carbohydrates in starches stimulate the sweet taste receptors on the tip of the tongue, where gastronomic pleasure begins. Eat enough starches

> *Starchy vegetables include:*
> *Grains:* barley, buckwheat, corn, millet, oats, rice, rye, sorghum, wheat, wild rice
> *Legumes:* beans, lentils, peas
> *Vegetables:* carrots, artichokes, parsnips, sweet potatoes, potatoes, winter squashes

and your body will release hormones and go through neurological changes that ensure long-term satisfaction."[49]

For those who just cannot believe that sweet potatoes are the real deal as nutritional powerhouses, try telling that to the Okinawans of Japan. They have the highest percentage of centenarians in the world, they have fewer metabolic and chronic diseases than we do in America, they're not overweight and they're full of energy. And, by the way, it just so happens that 69% of their calories are derived from sweet potatoes.[50] That is a high percentage from just one food, but it appears that long, long ago the Okinawans figured out something that Americans have not comprehended. If you want to substitute fruit with sweet potatoes in the morning, go right ahead and knock yourself out. It is far superior to bacon and eggs.

CALL TO ACTION

Goal: *Eat raw fruit for breakfast, as much as you want. Wait at least two hours before eating anything else.*

Raw fruit, raw nuts and water should be your go-to breakfast. Give it a shot for the next few weeks. If you feel you are falling off track, try a cooked, starchy vegetable. Baked potatoes or sweet potatoes are highly recommended.

If this step is at all difficult it will be because you are accustomed or addicted to something other than fruit. Many people get into a routine and do not want to make a change for the greater good. They wake up and eat oatmeal, yoghurt and drink organic milk because the media says those are the foods that are healthiest. Well, where has that philosophy taken us? I know plenty of overweight, unhealthy people who will swear to the virtues of oatmeal, yoghurt and organic milk. It is understood that most people will zealously defend their eating styles, but there's nothing better metabolically than the beautiful fruits nature has provided for us. Absolutely nothing! If you are eating so-called healthy foods and you feel out of shape, overweight or a lack of energy, then this should be a clear sign that something isn't right.

Many clients I have worked with believe they feel great eating "healthy" foods for breakfast, but that assessment is relative. Once they discover the power of fruit, they quickly reassess. It is difficult to understand how superior the fruit option is until you have tried it for a solid week or so. Remember, there is no good or bad food, only good or bad results. If you do not like your results, change your food.

Eat well and stay young!

If you're concerned about your health, you should probably avoid products that make health claims. Why? Because a health claim on a food product is a strong indication it's not really food, and food is what you want to eat.

Michael Pollan, In Defense of Food

Step 4 – The Green Leafy Hero

The green leafy vegetable is the champion of all foods. Pound for pound, green leafy vegetables are the best fighters we have against "olding". They have the power to save us from all types of metabolic issues, but they do not get much respect in American culture. They are not considered comfort food, nor are they considered satisfying and filling. Yet, if you fully embrace them in your eating style, odds are you will do far better than you could ever have imagined.

> *It is with great sadness and a heavy heart that I have to announce that I ate kale and liked it.*
> *– Greg Behrendt*

Leaves Are Not only to be Raked

Green leafy vegetables pack more nutrients per calorie than any other food we consume. Eating them is the key to staying young. Most are unaware of this fact because we have been conditioned to eat processed food that is "enriched" and "fortified" with all sorts of extracted and inferior vitamins and minerals. Then, when we think about someone eating green leafy vegetables, we wonder how can that person possibly be energetic and strong? Images of a weakling, barely able to do a push-up, come to mind. Who would think of green leafy vegetables being manly like a broiled steak, rack of lamb, Big Mac or Whopper? There are not any commercials I know of with a buff guy chomping on spinach and broccoli. At least we had Popeye cartoons back when I was a kid in the 60s, but those days are long gone. Someone was very wise way back then, but today Americans are getting sicker at accelerated rates and drugs do not provide the cure. Slowly, but surely, the tides are turning as many who are ill are seeking superior alternatives. Popeye and his cans of spinach are beginning to make sense again, as we have solid evidence that green leafy vegetables provide the metabolic power that we need.

Imitation Food

Our society has a twisted way of determining how we measure the nutritive content of food. We are conditioned to believe that we can add and subtract vitamins and minerals from food and it will become more powerful. "Fortification" and "enrichment" are marketing terms used to invoke feelings of power being added to what is being sold. However, those processes were necessary because there were vitamins and minerals stripped away during food processing. If some of those vitamins and minerals were not added back, we would have something denatured, unhealthy and possibly toxic.

> *About 80% of the food on shelves of supermarkets today didn't exist 100 years ago. – Larry McCleary*

Years ago, much of what was left behind during food processing was legally deemed to be unacceptable as food. Back in 1938, the Food, Drug and Cosmetic Act mandated that any food that was changed from its natural state must be labeled "imitation" food.[51] Of course, the food manufacturers fought against that labeling. Due to political pressure, that law has been disregarded since the 1970s. Alas, the food manufacturers got the green light they were hoping for. All they had to do was "fortify" or "enrich" the "imitation" food with vitamins and minerals, market it as healthy, and it could be sold for some serious profit. Hence, we have all sorts of food products, in beautiful packaging, which the public believes promotes health. Those food products are in the middle aisles of the supermarket and are to be limited or avoided. Remember that anything "fortified" or "enriched" is still imitation food which can do us great harm.

The "Jelly Bean Rule"

Years ago food manufacturers were free to put the word "healthy" on any product for marketing purposes. However, in 1994 the U.S. Food and Drug Administration began to enforce the "jelly bean rule". Its purpose was to protect consumers so they would not be duped or seduced by food labeling. Essentially, a food manufacturer cannot portray a product as "healthy" if it is low in fat, like a jelly bean, but has little to no additional nutritive value. The "jelly bean rule" states, "For a company to use the word healthy, or variations on it, like healthful, either in a brand name or as a descriptive term, the food must be low in fat and saturated fat and have limited amounts of sodium and cholesterol. The food must also contain at least 10 percent of the recommended daily value of one of the following: vitamin A, vitamin C, iron, calcium, protein or fiber. In most cases, those nutrients would have to occur naturally in the food."[52]

Has the "jelly bean rule" served the public well? My best guess is that it is similar to the argument of a mentholated cigarette being healthier than a regular cigarette. Neither option produces good results. That said, with the "jelly bean rule" being enforced, anything marketed as "healthy" must still be avoided and considered junk food. Of course, there is no need to be concerned regarding foods from the first aisle being marketed as "healthy". They contain no labels and fruits and vegetables in their natural state have always been proven to be health promoting.

Should We Weigh in?

Another way we are conditioned is to base nutrition on how much we eat instead of what we eat. We measure food with ounces, grams, cups and liters. We tend to think that, if we eat less, we will lose weight and be in better shape. That's nowhere near reality. If you eat less harmful food, you will probably feel hungry all the time and become malnourished. Eventually your discipline will splinter and you will satisfy that hunger by binging. It happens all the time unless you are extraordinarily disciplined, which 99% of people are not. However, when you eat certain types of food, such as green, leafy vegetables, you can eat as much as you want with basically no detrimental effects—except for maybe a bellyache from overeating. This method focuses your discipline from how much you eat to what you eat, which is the key to superior metabolic functioning.

To accentuate the point, of all the diet programs in America, Weight Watchers is the one I find the most intriguing. Participants are given points for eating certain types of food. The objective is to stay under a certain point limit for the day. About six years ago one of my clients ate too many cookies and exceeded her daily point total. She then said to me, "I guess all I can have is fruit the rest of the night. What a bummer!" She then explained that Weight Watchers does not give points for fruits and vegetables. I was floored. It sounds like they are saying fruits and vegetables may be eaten in unlimited quantities and there is no weight gain to be concerned about. It sounds like Raw Energy Vitality. (*However, to my dismay, Weight Watchers has changed its food policy as of last year. It now awards zero points to many foods that are not fruits and veggies.*)

The point is we are eating too much of the wrong foods, based on the options we allow to be placed before us. We are excessively consuming foods that are too calorically dense, stripped of nutrients, totally lacking fiber and loaded with salt, sugar, fat and toxic additives. To its credit, the processed food industry has found the perfect way to make it sexy so you will go wild when you see it. This cycle must be broken immediately for you to thwart the "olding" process. It is not that you should never have a potato chip, hot dog, corn chip or chocolate chip cookie; however, those foods should not be the foundation of your eating style when you have such an array of options available in this country. They must be consumed occasionally, if at all, and treated as "treats".

Where Do You Get Your Protein from?

> *The primary benefit of a vegan diet is that the removal of animal products usually necessitates a higher amount of nutrient-rich plant produce. The cons of a vegan diet could be the inclusion of too much heavily processed food, including seitan and isolated soy protein, flour, sweeteners and oils. – Joel Fuhrman, MD*

We are also way off base due to a lack of understanding of which vitamins and nutrients are in food. For instance, as mentioned in the previous chapter, we are too caught up in the hysteria of protein. "Where do you get your protein from?" has been asked of me a million times since adopting a vegan eating style in 1989. What people are really saying is "Vegetables do not have enough protein, so it is impossible to be healthy without eating meat." Of all the absurdities! That one question is proof positive that most people do not know what protein is, where it comes from, what foods contain it and/or how much is needed.

One of my stock answers to "Where do you get your protein from?" is to fire back another question: "How many people do you know who are suffering from a lack of protein?" This question usually invokes contemplative confusion because few people have thought about it. Sometimes I follow up with, "What disease or sickness do you get from a lack of protein?" Since 1989 I have never received an answer to those questions from a layperson. If you do not know what diseases you get from a lack of protein, nor do you know anyone who lacks sufficient protein in his or her diet, is there really a protein deficiency concern? The fact of the matter is that Americans get more protein than is necessary for optimal health. According to the National Center for Health Statistics, the average American gets twice as much as necessary.[53]

The more thoughtful question would be, "Do veggies contain enough protein to sustain a healthy life?" That question brings us to a major hurdle. You may have seen infomercials where huge piles of veggies are on a table. What follows is commentary such as "You must eat ALL of these vegetables to get the USDA recommended daily allowance of all your vitamins, nutrients and minerals." At that point the viewer is completely nonplussed. We can agree that we must eat more veggies for optimal health. But, as claimed by the infomercial and supposedly based on "research," you cannot possibly eat enough to be healthy. So you kill the idea of eating an ungodly number of veggies and buy a magic supplement to satisfy your mineral and nutrient deficiencies. If that is you, you are not alone; hence we now have a $37 billion vitamin supplement industry.[54] Metabolic syndrome, however, continues to rage out of control. The public is getting sicker and sicker because the magical supplements simply are not that magical.

Are Vitamin and Mineral Supplements the Answer?

The supplement industry needs serious investigation, as it is rife with malfeasance and controversy. No one knows definitively whether vitamin or mineral supplements work. Pieter A. Cohen, MD, wrote in an opinion article published in *JAMA (The Journal of the American Medical Association)*, "During the past 2 decades, a steady stream of high-quality studies evaluating dietary supplements has yielded predominantly disappointing results about potential health benefits, whereas evidence of harm has continued to accumulate. How consumers have responded to these scientific developments is not known."[55] A *New York Times* article by Liz Szabo of the Kaiser Health News references the opinions of Dr. Barnett Kramer, director of cancer prevention at the National Cancer Institute. In "Older Americans are 'Hooked' on Vitamins" Szabo wrote,

"A big part of the problem, Dr. Kramer said, could be that much nutrition research has been based on faulty assumptions, including the notion that people need more vitamins and minerals than a typical diet provides; that megadoses are always safe; and that scientists can boil down the benefits of vegetables like broccoli into a daily pill.

"Vitamin-rich foods can cure diseases related to vitamin deficiency. Oranges and limes were famously shown to prevent scurvy in vitamin-deprived 18th-century sailors. And research has long shown that populations that eat a lot of fruits and vegetables tend to be healthier than others.

"But when researchers tried to deliver the key ingredients of a healthy diet in a capsule, Dr. Kramer said, those efforts nearly always failed."[56]

Furthermore, it does not appear that the supplement industry is regulated sufficiently and many of the supplement manufacturers are getting away with murder. In a 2013 article, *The New York Times* found "DNA testing shows that many pills labeled as healing herbs are little more than powdered rice and weeds."[57]. After testing 44 different herbal supplement products, BMC (BioMed Centralwhich) Medicine found "Most of the herbal products tested were of poor quality, including considerable product substitution, contamination and use of fillers."[58]

Regardless of the duplicity of the supplement industry, it appears that the USDA recommended daily allowances are all overstated, misstated or misguided. For instance, as reported in a *Time* article by Alice Clark, "Study: U.S. Calcium Guidelines May Be Too High", the U.S. calcium recommendation is 1200mg per day for women over 50. However, that number has been refuted with claims that it may cause more bone fractures than preventing them.[59] The World Health Organization calcium guideline is only half as much as the USDA guideline. Such a wide disparity leads many to believe that the USDA guideline is influenced by industry desires rather than metabolic needs.

Supplement advertisements claim it is impossible to engage in a plant-based eating style and satisfy the USDA guidelines, while at the same time maintaining your vitality. If that is true, eating from the first aisle would be a total waste of time and we would be chasing our tails in the quest to be healthy. However, nature will not disappoint us! There is a surefire way to get the full quantity of necessary nutrients, not based on industry-influenced recommendations, but through simple observation and execution. I embraced veganism back in 1989 and transitioned to become a First Aisler, yet I have not suffered from any lack of nutrients on all my medical testing. My energy level is greater than most people I know in my age range. I am stronger and more balanced than most people I know in my age range. All of that is without paying any attention to the recommended daily allowances, while focusing on a plant-based diet by consuming green leafy veggies as much as possible. Is it possible that I am doing *something* right? Popular science and nutrition will probably say no, but when your body gives you positive feedback, it is wise to listen. And, according to my clients that follow my eating suggestions, they are experiencing positive gains as well.

Are Protein Powders the Answer?

The isolated protein-based supplements seem to have the desired effect of building muscle, but are they dangerous? Many people at my gym pour protein powders in their water

> *The most important thing to remember about food labels is that you should avoid foods that have labels. —* Joel Fuhrman, MD

bottles and shake up some type of colorful concoction every day. When I read the labels of those protein products I am thoroughly confused. It seems like a long list of dangerous chemicals whose harmful effects will only be detected once the consumer gets older. But, there are also immediate concerns.

About two years ago I worked with a 25-year-old guy who developed kidney failure due to ingesting too much protein powder. He was in the gym pumping iron like crazy. He was getting stronger and more muscular, exactly what he wanted. He looked phenomenal, but his kidneys needed some relief. Thankfully he was able to bounce back after a brief stint in the hospital.

A big problem is that excessive protein consumption raises the acidity level of your blood. I had another client who engaged in a highly acidic diet, rife with processed food and animal products. On top of that, he added protein supplements to burn fat and build muscle. His method failed as he developed kidney stones. He had to endure excruciating pain in the hospital for three days, followed by weeks of home recovery. Adding protein supplements to an already highly acidic diet is a recipe for disaster, so proceed with caution if you dare to use them.

Which Green Leaves Are Best?

ANDI Chart

1. Kale
2. Collard Greens
3. Mustard Greens
4. Watercress
5. Swiss Chard
6. Bok Choy
7. Spinach
8. Arugula
9. Romaine
10. Brussel Sprouts

By introducing raw salads into your life, you will take the most serious stride of REV. There is no doubt it will increase the upward trajectory of your energy levels, reduce your stress levels and keep you younger. On the ANDI (Aggregate Nutrient Density Index) chart developed by Joel Fuhrman, MD and author of *Eat to Live*, green, leafy veggies are the most nutrient dense foods on the planet. That means, per calorie, they give you the most vitamins, minerals and phytochemicals that you can get from any food. They dominate the top 10 foods on the ANDI chart.[60] By adding the raw salad to your eating style, replete with green, leafy veggies, you will ascend to the peak of the nutritional mountain! Dr. Fuhrman's equation for nutritional excellence is:

$$H = N/C \quad (Health = Nutrients / Calories)$$

If you believe in what Dr. Fuhrman is reporting, shouldn't you eat more of the nutrient dense foods than any others? This method does seem to make sense if you want the most bang for your buck nutritionally. Of course, from time to time we must incorporate all the other colorful veggies into our salad bowls because they also pack a powerful punch. As an added benefit, what you are really doing, without thinking about it, is giving yourself a special gift whose power should never be underestimated: superior digestion through the magic of fiber. This was done by the introduction of more fruit into your system in the previous stage, but now we are taking it to a higher level.

Fiber is the Magic Ingredient

Fiber is something we seem to gloss over when we eat food. Like all other vitamins, minerals and nutrients, it is something we cannot see, but we understand its value. The older folks I have known would talk about being "regular," meaning they wanted better bowel movements. Upon reflection, I am not sure they had the best approach. Most of them got a doctor's prescription to smooth things out. Others ended up dashing to the store to purchase products like Benefiber, Metamucil or FiberSmart. Today, those who deem themselves more "sophisticated" go for the natural psyllium husks. None of those options compare to eating more fruits and veggies. Actually, they are a complete waste of time if you continue to consume the same food that caused constipation in the first place. As Dr. Joel Fuhrman would say, lazy and undisciplined people want to "buy health in a bottle." It is time to rethink that philosophy.

> *The answer isn't another pill. The answer is spinach. — Bill Maher*

It is heartbreaking to think about how many of us are dealing with digestion and constipation issues. In 2010, 60-70 million Americans were suffering with digestive diseases.[61] That is not counting those who do not go to the doctor or emergency room because of a bellyache. It is also not counting those for whom constipation becomes the norm and they do not even realize they are constipated. They just deal with it in silent agony.

At the gym, I see men go to the toilet for a little "recreational defecation." They are sitting on the throne for seemingly an eternity, sending texts, reading the *Wall Street Journal*, dealing with office issues, etc. Once one gentleman processed his bowel movement, but stood outside the stall of his friend for another 10 minutes to finish their conversation. It cannot be too pretty when you need that much time to release fecal matter. Another time I saw a pair of sneakers under a stall as I went to the shower. I came back as clean as a whistle

> *Societies that eat unrefined foods produce large stools and build small hospitals; societies that eat fiber-depleted foods produce small stools and build large hospitals. — Denis Parsons Burkitt*

20 minutes later and I saw the same pair of sneakers under the same stall. That is a serious problem!

The solution is so simple and easy. Something very interesting happens to your body when more fiber is introduced, via whole, plant-based foods. Your digestion and bowel movements miraculously get smoother. Of course, it is not a miracle, but you get the point. In the previous scenarios, if those people just increased fruit and veggie consumption, along with water consumption, I would bet that 95% of their digestive problems would begin to clear up within 24 to 72 hours. This has happened countless times with many different clients. They are literally shocked by the simplicity of the solution.

For the record, I would say if you eat a proper amount of fiber-rich food and drink plenty of water, you would have at least three bowel movements per day. One per meal should be about average. That statement shocks most people I know, thinking that only one a day is optimal. I would go on to say, if you only have one per day—or less—there is a serious problem. You are just asking for a metabolic disease to burgeon and wreak havoc on your body.

It's Gut Check Time!

Years ago I had two clients who suffered with Inflammatory Bowel Disease (IBD), a combination of Crohn's disease and/or ulcerative colitis. It can be a painful and mentally devastating autoimmune disorder. It can also be exacerbated by a high percentage of fiber-less foods; basically, highly processed foods, including meats and dairy products, which are not whole fruits, veggies and grains. Those two clients went back and forth from one doctor to another getting all types of pharmaceutical concoctions, none of which cured the disease (actually, there is no known cure) and all of which had stressful side effects. I recommended simply eating more fruits and salads. Unfortunately, with IBD, eating raw fruits and/or veggies can be an irritant for some, but oftentimes moderate amounts are helpful, along with cooked veggies. When those clients followed my recommendations, both said their abdominal pain eased. It was not a cure, but it was a major improvement.

> If beef is your idea of 'real food for real people,' you'd better live real close to a real good hospital. – Neal Barnard, MD

One of my aunts was on the swine and chicken embryo breakfast plan (affectionately known as bacon and eggs) for most of her life, followed by other animal flesh products for lunch. As aforementioned, there is no good or bad food, only desirable or undesirable results. Every day, however, her result was pain. She even had to be hospitalized a few times, as she suffered from diverticulitis. Her bowels were on lockdown as her doctors prescribed medication after medication, none of which worked for her. Unfortunately, I found out when she was 70 years old that she had been suffering for the past 15 to 20 years. I begged her to drink more water and start eating fruit for breakfast and a salad for lunch. As an enticement, she reluctantly bought in when I compromised and said, "You can still have your bacon and eggs, but save it for lunch, only after you've eaten your salad." Within a few days of following my advice, her bowels started flowing like a river and her pain subsided. She was shocked by the improvement, but it was bound to happen. When you put the right kind of fiber in your system—not fiber bars, but fruits and veggies—everything seems to flow.

If your diet is bereft of those simple foods, those that fell off a tree or popped out of the ground, you will most likely suffer from some type of digestive disorder. The disorder can sometimes be painful and messy, like diverticulitis, which is caused by excessive straining to move fecal matter through your intestines. Polyps then develop on the small intestine and the result can be bloody stool, cramping and pain. Or the disorder could be indirectly painful, such as developing a leaky gut where noxious proteins or microbes seep into your bloodstream and invade your body. They wreak havoc and the result can be maladies such as cancer, type 2 diabetes, high blood pressure and cardiovascular disease. To those with a leaky gut, it is impossible to know if the increased fruit and veggie consumption is doing the job in all cases, but everyone feels better as the antioxidants, minerals and other phytochemicals begin the healing process. Regardless of how your intestinal problems manifest, greater fruit and veggie consumption is a stress reliever and an energy increaser.

Raw Salad or Cooked Food?

Many people eat salad every day, but their salads are toxic. They add exotic cheeses, meats, poultry, fish, oils, dressings and who knows what else to a few leaves, then ordain it as a healthy meal. But, at this stage of REV, we know better. The power of raw veggies in your salad is that cooking has not altered the chemical composition of your food, nor does adding non-plant products dilute the power. Many in the raw food community believe that heating veggies above 110 degrees Fahrenheit changes the nature of the veggies and destroys their enzymes, potentially making them harmful to the system. To the contrary, others argue that the rapid mental growth of man is due to foods being cooked that release certain enzymes. There is no consensus on which theory is more likely or true, if not both. But, at this point, it does not make a difference which side is more accurate because today's stats show that only 7-8% of our calories are derived from fruits and vegetables. That minute percentage is not working metabolically for Americans. We need more raw food to balance the scales.

Some veggies appear to be more fun to eat cooked, while others are great cooked or raw. Broccoli or kale does not thrill me raw, but steamed or sautéed I love them. I have yet to eat a raw sweet potato and have no plans to do so; but when it is baked I cannot get enough. What really matters is increasing your raw food consumption to raise your energy level, reduce stress and stay young, not to prove a point by going totally raw (although that's fine if you prefer it). If you feel you must have some cooked or non-plant foods for lunch, go right ahead and knock yourself out. However, at least try to eat a raw salad first for the next few weeks. You will be pleasantly surprised!

Acid/Alkaline Ratio

One of the beauties of eating raw foods is that they make it easier for the body's acid/alkaline ratio to be in optimal balance. The human body functions optimally when blood pH is between 7.35 to 7.45. The acidic promoting foods that the average American eats makes it more taxing on the body to maintain that range. When digesting those foods—such as processed flours, meats, cheeses, oils and all the "comfort foods" Americans have become so

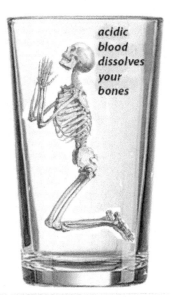

acidic blood dissolves your bones

discomforted by—the body's metabolism must work harder to keep the blood pH from falling below 7.35 into metabolic acidosis. That extra work results in exhaustion of the body's mineral reserves. When your blood is too acidic, it uses calcium to neutralize the acid and raise your blood pH. If you do not get enough calcium from the food you eat, it's leached from your bones. It is like dipping your skeleton in a glass of acid for years on end and it's begging to get out. The excessive acid increases the odds of developing osteoporosis, osteopenia, kidney stones, arthritis or something similarly undesirable.

Industrialized nations that consume high amounts of processed and meat-based foods have higher rates of osteoporosis and hip fractures, due to bone loss. Following is the InsiderMonkey.com list of *11 Countries with Highest Rates of Osteoporosis in the World.*[62]

Highest Rates of Osteoporosis in the World

1. United States
2. United Kingdom
3. Sweden
4. Finland
5. China
6. Russia
7. Brazil
8. Australia
9. Canada
10. Germany
11. France

Years ago I worked with a personal trainer who was absolutely convinced that osteopenia ran in her family. I opined that yes, genetically it is possible your family has a higher susceptibility to contract osteopenia; but have you ever considered investigating the eating patterns of your family? Is everyone eating lots of meat, dairy, cheeses and processed foods? She thought about it for a moment and confessed her family did just that. Unfortunately, she could not see the connection between that type of eating style and osteopenia. She thought that taking calcium supplements would help her family members, but that solution was not working too well.

An important fact to remember is that all natural diets, including purely vegetarian diets without a hint of dairy products, contain amounts of calcium that are above the threshold for meeting your nutritional needs... In fact, calcium deficiency caused by an insufficient amount of calcium in the diet is not known to occur in humans. – John McDougall

Most people believe drinking milk and taking calcium supplements solve the calcium loss problem, but those methods may actually do more harm than good. The bottom line is that it does not matter how much milk, supplements or drugs we ingest because it is impossible to intake enough calcium to counter how much we lose, due to eating acid forming foods. In a September 2015 article, *Today.com* reported "The findings, reported in the *British Medical Journal's* online publication *BMJ.com*, support what U.S. health officials have been telling Americans for a few years now—taking calcium supplements is not just a waste of time, but it could be harmful. The extra calcium does not go to strengthen bones but instead can build up in the arteries, causing heart disease, or in the kidneys, causing kidney stones."[63] I have been telling people that same thing since 1989, yet few would listen to me. Oh well…

Can eating alkaline based foods help solve the calcium loss problem? Absolutely! By eating alkalinizing foods your body does not need to extract as much from the mineral reserves in your bones to lower your blood acid level. Additionally, raw vegetables have a much higher calcium ratio per calorie than processed foods or meat products. Consequently, you are extracting less bone calcium while ingesting a sufficient amount through the food you eat. It is easy to see that raw vegetables can safeguard you from a calcium deficiency.

Following is a short list of foods that have an alkalinizing effect on the body:

Alkaline Vegetables*: Beets, Broccoli, Cauliflower, Celery, Cucumber, Kale, Lettuce, Onions, Peas, Peppers, Spinach*

Alkaline Fruits*: Apple, Banana, Berries, Cantaloupe, Grapes, Melon, Lemon, Orange, Peach, Pear, Watermelon*

Alkaline Nuts*: Almonds, Chestnuts, Tofu*

Alkaline Spices*: Cinnamon, Curry, Ginger, Mustard, Sea Salt*

(To clear any confusion, the pH scale goes from 0 to 14. The acid range is below 7; the alkaline range is above 7; and 7 is neutral. If a food is acidic on the pH scale, it does not necessarily mean it has an acidic affect on the body. For instance, lemons are acidic on the pH scale, yet have an alkalinizing effect on the body, once the citric acid in them is metabolized. Cooked fruits and veggies are usually alkaline also, as they would be when they are raw. However, once we start adding condiments and oils, those are usually acidic.)

Take Your Vitamins

> *Everything in food works together to create health or disease. The more we think that a single chemical characterizes a whole food, the more we stray into idiocy. —*
> *T. Colin Campbell*

Raw fruits and veggies in your salad also provide the best source of vitamins and minerals. The average American thinks he can add vitamins and minerals to his diet by going to a health food store and buying supplements. That is the lazy and ineffective way. Back in 1933, vitamin C was the first vitamin to be synthesized (a process invented by Dr. Tadeusz Reichstein, of the Swiss Institute of Technology in Zurich). With that discovery it was not long before vitamins were bottled, sold, and touted as panaceas for all our dietary indiscretions. Coincidentally, since the sale of vitamins has risen, so have the rates of cancer and other diseases. It appears that those same vitamins, once processed and bottled, are not defending us as we might think.

Many in the scientific community believe that vitamin and mineral supplements are a total waste of time based on research published in 2013.[64] One reason could be that, when vitamins are isolated, they do not pack the same punch as they do when combined with other vitamins, minerals and phytochemicals, as nature intended. For instance, you can take all the calcium supplements in the world, but if your vitamin D is insufficient, the calcium may not be absorbed. Currently dieticians, food scientists and nutritionists do not fully understand the relationships among the thousands of phytochemicals, vitamins and minerals in plants. Human ingenuity is simply not that advanced, but fortunately, nature can rescue us from the human arrogance of believing we know more than we do. It has perfected those relationships for our benefit. There may be no great need for isolated supplements in a bottle, in lieu of simply eating your veggies. I have many clients who swear by vitamins, but I always admonish them to eat their fruits and veggies first. If that is done, additional vitamin supplements may have a chance to add some benefit.

Bulk Up Your Salad

Eating a raw salad, rife with green leafy veggies, root veggies and fruit will certainly put you on an upward trajectory health-wise. However, if you feel you must have a little more bulk or variety in your salad to ease your transition into plant-based eating, I would recommend starchy vegetables. John McDougall, MD, is famous for saying, "Archeological research shows that starches have been the primary food source throughout the world for 5,000 to 10,000 years, or even longer."[65] To the best of my knowledge, he is absolutely correct; and I have not heard anyone refute that assertion. Worldwide, different areas of the globe thrive on certain starches.

Corn (maize) – North, Central and South America for 7,000 years

Potatoes – South America (Andes) for 13,000 years

Legumes – America, Asia and Europe for 6,000 years

Sweet Potatoes – South America and Caribbean for 5,000 years

Millet – Africa for 6,000 years

Sorghum – East Africa for 6,000 years

Barley – Middle East for 11,000 years

Oats – Middle East for 11,000 years

Wheat – Near East for 10,000 years

Rice – Asia for 10,000 years

Rye – Asia for 5,000 years

So, if your raw salad needs a little help, I am a big believer that including starchy vegetables is not a bad idea. They provide a slower burn for sustained energy and they also give you a feeling of fullness. When I was fortunate enough to attend one of Dr. McDougall's multi-day events, everybody was packing in the starches and having a ball. The food was great.

My favorite starch is quinoa (technically it's a seed, not a grain). It originated in the Andes and many in that region believe it gives you more power than potatoes. One of my clients from Peru almost burst into joyful tears when I told her to include a little quinoa in her lunchtime salad if she cared to. Coming to the U.S.A. she had practically forgotten about how filling and nutritious quinoa is. I also like corn, potatoes, legumes and millet in my salad, but be very careful how they are prepared. Oftentimes salad bars sneak in all kinds of unhealthy stuff and the starchy veggie can become toxic. Include them in your salad without anything else added. Also, if you have gluten sensitivity, then stay away from barley, rye and wheat.

CALL TO ACTION

Objective: *Eat a large, raw salad for lunch every day, filled with lots of green, leafy vegetables.*

Your challenge is quite simple. Remember, stages one through three are still in effect. Continue to drink plenty of water, eat six pieces of fruit per day and refrain from eating anything but fruit for breakfast. But now, in stage four, we must add the power of green, leafy vegetables to your eating regimen. Your mission is to eat a large, raw salad for lunch every day, filled with lots of green, leafy vegetables. Go wild with any combination of romaine lettuce, kale, spinach, bok choy, mustard greens, etc. Throw in any veggies or fruits that make it more delectable, such as tomatoes, cucumbers, grapes, oranges, mushrooms, carrots or beets. Add any spices you like, such as basil, oregano, dill or parsley. Believe it or not, this is the biggest step you will ever take toward superior health and maximization of your metabolic energy.

The best salad would be the one you prepare at home, but labor intensity may be an issue. I used to visit salad bars way too often, but convenience is the name of the game when you live a fast-paced life. At a salad bar my salad oftentimes weighs in at more than 1.5 lbs. That would probably be far more than necessary to fill you up. When my clients do this for a week or more they have reported feeling much lighter in the abdominal area and more energized. Stuff as much salad into your body as possible. Then, opt for oil-free and low sodium dressings if nothing natural is available.

My favorite salad dressings are the ones I make at home. Take any nut (I prefer pecans), any fruit (I prefer oranges, blueberries, apples) and raw apple cider vinegar. Put them into a blender and you will have a beautiful, creamy salad dressing. If you cannot tolerate nuts, try quinoa instead. Another great blender combination is avocado, cucumber, vinegar or lemon juice and a bulb of garlic. It's heavenly!

I strongly urge you to buy a cookbook to prepare raw or vegan salad dressings and marinades. The combinations are endless and most ingredients can be found right in the first aisle of the supermarket.

The green, leafy veggie reigns supreme!

Regardless of whether we are required to purchase medical insurance, know that we can only buy real health insurance in the produce section of the local supermarket.

Joel Fuhrman, MD

Step 5 – Dinner Time is the Best Time

At this point you may be quite tired of all this talk about raw food—and I cannot blame you! Breakfast was fruit and lunch was salad. Your body is extremely pleased that you are giving it an abundance of vitamins, minerals and fiber, but now you may be ready for something charbroiled, sautéed, steamed and maybe even burned to a crisp. Much to your delight, REV dinner-time is a most interesting time of day because your focus will no longer be solely on raw food. Cooked food is a lot of fun and nutritious, so we may as well take advantage of it.

Should We Cook Food?

Many in the raw food community believe problems arise when food is cooked, partly due to research conducted by Dr. Paul Kouchakoff in the 1930s. He found that there is a rise in white blood cells when food is eaten that has been cooked above certain temperatures, approximately 110 degrees Fahrenheit, a process called digestive leukocytosis. However, Dr. Kouchakoff believed that digestive leukocytosis can be neutralized by eating raw food with your cooked food.[66] There is not much documentation regarding subsequent studies to corroborate his findings, but chemical reactions obviously occur when food is heated. Enzymes, minerals and vitamins can be altered or destroyed. For instance, vitamin C and potassium do not survive the cooking process. Yet, there are many foods that may be enhanced by cooking. The antioxidants in carrots, tomatoes and peppers are released when cell walls are broken down by heat.[67] In addition, there are many foods that must be cooked to ease the digestive process. Who wants to live in a world without steamed rice or baked potatoes? Can you imagine being served a cold and blood drenched steak on your plate? (*Actually, I know some people who say they do, but that's just a little too ambitious for me.*) Cooking has a firm grip in all cultures and excluding it from the eating process is an impossible undertaking.

REV is about expanding your raw fruit and vegetable intake, not excluding cooked food. Cooked veggies, grains and fruits are to be embraced and enjoyed, but we must be aware of any potential dangers of the cooking process. The Hippocrates Health Institute in Palm Beach, Florida, promotes a raw vegan lifestyle to combat the perils of cooked food consumption. Some of the toxic substances produced when food is cooked and/or processed have been shown to accelerate aging and promote diseases, such as cancer. For instance, heating starchy carbohydrates like breads and potatoes, produces acrylamides. When meat is grilled and charred, polycyclic hydrocarbons are formed. (*See Appendix F – The Perils of Cooked Food*). It appears that all forms of cooking food produce some type of undesirable side effect, accentuating the need to consume more raw produce to counter the cooking process.

Which Cooking Method is Least Harmful

Since we are going to consume cooked food, what cooking method is the best or least harmful? The basic cooking methods are: Deep-Fry, Pan-Fry, Stir-Fry, Grill, Broil,

Sautee, Roast, Bake, Sear, Poach, Simmer, Boil, Steam, Blanch, Braise, Stew.

For me, steaming appears to be the safest and easiest method for cooking vegetables. It preserves the integrity of the vegetables more than the other methods since there is only steam contacting them at a temp of 100C (212F). No oil or foreign substance is necessary to aid the cooking process and the vegetables do not release any nutrients into a liquid like water. It is quick and easy, ten minutes or so in most cases.

Baking is also a great method for cooking all types of potatoes, as sweet potatoes are one of my favorite foods. You can wrap them up and toss them in the oven for an hour or so. As with steaming, you do not need any oils or substances to complete the cooking process.

Simmering and boiling are obviously great for cooking bean and vegetable soups. I am a big fan of lentils, split peas, black-eye peas, black beans, adzuki, and chickpeas. There's nothing more joyous than combining your favorite beans, veggies and spices in a pot and having a soup party.

Be careful ordering vegetable soup when you are out on the town. Many chefs add chicken or beef stock to vegetable soups to "enhance" flavor. Those who add it do not really know about enhancing flavor without the use of those stocks, which is sad and frustrating for many who desire to go fully plant-based. Most of those stocks are loaded with sodium (as are vegetable stocks), even when they tout "low sodium". Unfortunately, many cooks cannot operate without them and never enjoy all plant-based soups. If you must, add your salt after your food is cooked, not during the cooking process.

Deep-frying and pan-frying are best to be limited or avoided completely, as fried foods are extremely taxing on the body. Of course, Kentucky Fried Chicken would not agree, but the amount of saturated fat in fried foods increases your risk for cholesterol and heart problems, with certain types of cancer and obesity lurking in the bushes.

What Type of Protein Would You Like?

> *Every time you eat or drink, you are either feeding disease or fighting it. – Heather Morgan, MS, NLC*

Now that we have introduced cooked food into the process, it is fair to assume that you may want some meat on the dinner menu. Or do you want protein on the dinner menu? While visiting my family during the Christmas season, we went to a salad buffet restaurant. Near the end of the buffet line, the server asked me, "What type of protein would you like in your salad?" The options were chicken, fish, beef or tofu. Of course, the server had no clue regarding the protein content in green veggies, as she was simply doing her job.

Incessant advertising and government lobbying has painted the picture that only animal products contain sufficient amounts of protein for humans to thrive. After almost three decades of plant-based eating, I have had countless, highly intelligent people ask me, "Where do you get your protein from?" They had absolutely no idea there were adequate amounts of protein in vegetables.

Even more alarming is that many people are now saying they desire protein, not meat, as if you can interchange the two. Meat has received some negative press in this country, but protein has been praised and reigns supreme among nutrients. Mostly everyone raves about protein and wants more. That being acknowledged, we must credit the meat and dairy industries for pulling off one the greatest marketing campaigns in history: they have effectively married the words "meat" and "protein," thereby removing any stigma of meat consumption from the minds of those at the dinner table. The sentiment is, forget about the evidence that meat consumption is linked to cancer and heart disease, meat has protein in it, so it must be good. It is an unparalleled marketing strategy—nothing short of brilliant—but metabolically devastating.

The Food Plate Deception

The message that only meat and dairy products contain protein is never directly stated by the food industry or media because that would be a flat out lie, but subliminally it is implanted all over the place. On the current government sponsored Food Plate, you'll notice that protein is the only macronutrient which has its own section. Carbohydrates and fats are just as important as protein, yet they are not represented on the Food Plate; and dairy is such a darling that it has its own mini plate.

The Food Plate would lead you to believe that fruits, vegetables and grains contain no protein and you "must" get it from a special source to be healthy. Wonder what that special source could be? By now you know the answer.

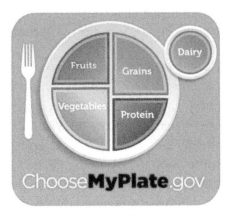

That's Too Much Protein

That fact is Americans consume way too much protein and we suffer because of it. The average American gets approximately 30% of his calories from protein, mostly derived from meat and dairy products. On top of that, I see far too many gym rats pumping protein shakes into their bodies to get "big". As mentioned in the previous chapter, excessive protein raises the acidity of your blood, leading to kidney issues, arthritis, gout attacks, etcetera.

The question is how do we cut down our protein intake to a reasonable level? The average American male consumes about 102 grams of protein per day, while the average female consumes about 70 grams. It is almost twice as much as recommended by the Food and Nutrition Board.[68] The key to more reasonable protein levels—also fat and carbohydrate levels—is to consume more fruits and veggies. Eating greater quantities of fruits and veggies, cooked and raw, will balance your carbohydrate, protein and fat ratios to more nature-designed levels, which are optimal levels for an energy-filled life. Taxing your digestive system with too much of one macronutrient will do nothing but make you grow older at a faster rate. Therefore, my best advice is to limit meat products as much as possible. One of my heroes, Michael Pollan, gives sound advice on the cover of *In Defense of Food*: "Eat food. Not too much. Mostly plants."

Beware of Animal Protein

Protein sources and quality for human consumption is something completely glossed over by the mainstream media and the public. There has been evidence that certain amino acids feed cancerous tumors, particularly methionine. According to Tina Kaczor, ND, FABNO, Editor-in-Chief of Natural Journal of Medicine, "There is direct evidence that methionine restriction leads to selective death of cancer cells versus normal cells."[69] It appears that cancer cells need methionine to grow and rarely, if ever, does mainstream media address that issue.

Dr. Michael Gregor, author of *How Not to Die* and blogger of NutrionFacts.org, wrote, "Forty years ago, a landmark paper was published showing for the first time that many human cancers have what's called 'absolute methionine dependency,' meaning that if we try to grow cells in a Petri dish without giving them the amino acid methionine, normal cells thrive, but without methionine, cancer cells die. Normal breast cells grow no matter what, with or without methionine, but cancer cells need that added methionine to grow."[70]   The problem is that methionine is a sulphur-containing amino acid (along with cysteine) and cancer needs extra sulphur to proliferate. It's shocking that this was known more than 40 years ago, yet you don't hear much about adopting a methionine restricted eating regimen.   Maybe that is because foods highest in methionine include beef, chicken, eggs, cheese, and dairy.[71] So not only are we consuming too much protein in general, we're also consuming dangerous levels of sulphur-containing amino acids, via meat products. It is no wonder we're "olding" at an accelerated rate.   Yet, as aforementioned, the solution is simple: more fruits and more veggies. Those are the foods lowest in methionine and highest in life promoting nutrients and minerals that fight cancer cells.

> Cow's milk protein may be the single most significant chemical carcinogen to which humans are exposed.
>
> T. Colin Campbell, MD

Just as dangerous is the amount of IGF-1 (insulin-like growth factor one) contained in animal products, especially dairy. The purpose of IGF-1 is to make animals grow during infancy.   But please keep in mind that a cow's milk is to grow a baby calf, not a human being. Cows naturally grow at a much faster rate than humans. A newborn calf doubles in size in approximately 45 days, while a newborn human child doubles in size in approximately 180 days. For a calf to grow at that rate it would need much more protein and IGF-1 than human milk can provide, hence cow's milk contains approximately three times the amount of protein than human milk. The real problem is that excessive dairy and IGF-1 consumption also promotes the growth of cancer cells.[72]

Green Leafy Veggies Contain the Best Protein

Regarding the confusion regarding the amounts of protein in vegetables versus animal products, let's see if we can clear it up a bit. Since most people are caught up in calorie consumption, as well as amounts of protein, we will start there. So, let us determine the amount of protein, in grams, based on the number of calories consumed. For instance, using information from Self Nutrition Data (http://nutritiondata.self.com/) we will compare protein, carb and fat amounts based on consuming the same number of calories of steak versus spinach. Unfortunately, I have not found a calculator to

> *In the next ten years, one of the things you're bound to hear is that animal protein is one of the most toxic nutrients of all that can be considered. Quite simply, the more you substitute plant foods for animal foods, the healthier you are likely to be.*
> *— T. Colin Campbell*

give you those numbers based on "calories consumed." We must do a little math to make the comparison work.

Steak
http://nutritiondata.self.com/facts/beef-products/6178/2

Nutrition Facts
Serving Size 1 ounce 28g (1 ounce (28g))

Amount Per Serving

Calories 45	Calories from Fat 14

	% Daily Value*
Total Fat 2g	2%
Saturated Fat 1g	3%
Trans Fat	
Cholesterol 18mg	6%
Sodium 20mg	1%
Total Carbohydrate 0g	0%
Dietary Fiber 0g	0%
Sugars 0g	
Protein 7g	

Vitamin A	0%	•	Vitamin C	0%
Calcium	0%	•	Iron	5%

*Percent Daily Values are based on a 2,000 calorie diet. Your daily values may be higher or lower depending on your calorie needs.

© www.NutritionData.com

Spinach
http://nutritiondata.self.com/facts/vegetables-and-vegetable-products/2626/2

Nutrition Facts
Serving Size 100 grams (100 grams)

Amount Per Serving

Calories 23	Calories from Fat 3

	% Daily Value*
Total Fat 0g	1%
Saturated Fat 0g	0%
Trans Fat	
Cholesterol 0mg	0%
Sodium 79mg	3%
Total Carbohydrate 4g	1%
Dietary Fiber 2g	9%
Sugars 0g	
Protein 3g	

Vitamin A	188%	•	Vitamin C	47%
Calcium	10%	•	Iron	15%

*Percent Daily Values are based on a 2,000 calorie diet. Your daily values may be higher or lower depending on your calorie needs.

© www.NutritionData.com

Using the spinach label, we must double the number of calories to approximately equal the same number of calories on the steak label. For example, if we double 23 calories of spinach we get 46 calories. We can then compare that against the 45 calories of steak (it's not exact, but close enough). Then, if we double the amount of protein from spinach, we get 6 grams versus 7 grams from the steak. This shows that if you consume equal amounts of calories of spinach and steak, you get about the same amount of protein from each food. If we go a little further, we can look at the numbers for carbohydrates, fats and other nutrients.

STEAK – 45 calories	SPINACH – 46 calories
Protein – 7 grams	Protein – 6 grams
Fat – 2 grams	Fat – 0 grams
Carbohydrates – 0 grams	Carbohydrates – 8 grams
Fiber – 0 grams	Fiber – 5 grams
Cholesterol – 18 mg	Cholesterol – 0 mg
Sodium – 20 mg	Sodium – 158 mg
Potassium – 82 mg	Potassium – 334 mg
Calcium – 2.2 mg	Calcium – 60 mg
Total Weight – 28 grams	Total Weight – 200 grams

Most people are shocked to see that spinach contains any protein at all and I implore you to fact check these numbers. Basically, the same amount of protein is in each food, provided you consume 45 to 46 calories of each food. The more startling number in the table is the total grams of food you can consume. Consuming 45 to 46 calories of each food, you can eat approximately seven times as much spinach as steak (200g of spinach vs. 28g of steak). Looking at the calcium and potassium numbers, you get much more from spinach than steak. There is no cholesterol in spinach and there is plenty of fiber. Spinach has steak beat in every way. It is obvious that a lot of calories are packed into a tiny amount of steak. With that understanding, you would have to eat a greater amount of steak to be satisfied; consequently, you would have a greater tendency to overeat. The danger is that you would consume too much protein and too many calories, which is precisely what most Americans do and why metabolic syndrome is raging. By eating spinach, you would have far fewer health concerns, if any at all. Obviously Popeye knew what he was doing!

The bottom line of this analysis is that you can eat a lot of green, leafy veggies. You would never have to worry about that feeling of hunger or starvation associated with most diets, nor would you have to be concerned about restricting your calories. It is damn near impossible to over-consume calories by eating lots of green, leafy veggies, not to mention all the additional nutrients and vitamins you would get that are bereft in animal products.

You are getting much more bang for your buck which is why REV works so beautifully regarding weight loss.

CALL TO ACTION

Objective: ***Fill half of your dinner plate with cooked veggies.***

Now it is time to chow down. You mission is for at least half of your dinner plate to be cooked veggies, whatever you enjoy the most. The other half is yours to play with. Many of my clients relish this time of day because they can consider steak, lamb chops, pork, cheeses; the things we love so much which cause so much strife.

By now you are fully aware of the power of fruits and veggies. You know what should be the preponderance of your daily food intake to be full of life. Think of meat products, desserts and highly processed foods as treats, not the foundation of your eating style. If you do so, they will not cause as much of a devastating effect and you will enjoy them much more.

Dine with pleasure!

The Gods created certain kinds of beings to replenish our bodies; they are the trees and the plants and the seeds.

Plato

Go All In!

Is a first aisle eating style the best way to go? It should be obvious by now, but if it is not, the answer is YES. I have been raving about it since 1989. It is fun, easy, energizing and maybe lifesaving for some. However, with all its magnificent virtues, it is not for everyone. We live in a meat-based society and that will not change anytime soon. We are so caught up in animal flesh and dairy that food manufacturers jump through hoops to make veggies taste like meat. Once I went to a French vegan restaurant and every dish was traditional French fare. I had coq au vin made with pea protein; and escargot made from mushrooms. They tasted wonderful, but for those who eat the animal product versions, I am sure they would pale in comparison. Personally, I do not need to be reminded of the animal products I decided to eschew back in 1989. That said, this chapter is only for those who truly want to cut meat products out of their lives, but just have not crossed the finish line yet. It breaks through all the rationalizations and excuses I have encountered in the last 29 years and gives you the wings to fly through the plant-based world.

If you have gone through the five steps of REV, you are far ahead of the great majority of Americans. Even if you stopped at step one, two, three or four, the benefits are still profound and you should be pleased. Ask your family and friends if they drink at least two quarts of water daily? Do they eat at least six pieces of fruit per day? Do they predominantly eat fruit for breakfast? Do they eat a large, raw salad daily? Is their dinner plate full of veggies, with meat products at a minimum? My best guess is that 99%

of those you ask will say no. If you have answered yes to any of those questions, you deserve a round of applause.

Going all in will give you the energy burst you need not only to survive, but also to thrive! If you do not believe that is true, after experiencing the first five stages, it is understandable. Most people are hesitant to commit to a first aisle eating style, for any duration, because they still believe meat-based products have some "magical" quality the vegetable world cannot touch. There is plenty of evidence to the contrary, but most people do not want to hear it. If you are one who shares that belief, the advertisers and media have seduced you. You have been sold a bogus bill of goods.

Get to the Source!

The meat and dairy industries are extremely powerful, and clever. Their marketing campaigns can make the average American believe almost anything about their products. The reality is that there is nothing in the animal kingdom that the plant kingdom does not possess in abundance and in higher quality. All the great things you hear about meat and dairy, if you hear anything at all, generate from the plant kingdom. Animals eat plants, or they eat other animals that eat plants, and those plants grow from the ground. Therefore, we must make a diligent effort to get to the source.

One hundred percent plant-based eating goes against the norm and it may always be a challenge to maintain your

eating integrity. There are many who I have spoken with about converting for years before they acted, but it is always a bad idea to rush any process. All you need for a successful transition is knowledge, discipline and the earth. The bottom line is that if you never eat animal products again, you will not miss a thing.

You Are Elite!

Imagine marathoners poised to compete. They are all packed together waiting for the starting gun to fire. At that moment, everyone is equal and tied for first place. The gun then fires and everyone is off and running. But, what happens as the race progresses? You quickly see that everyone is not equal, as an "elite" group breaks away and leads the pack. And, as the kilometers pile on, that elite group gets smaller and smaller. By engaging in a first aisle eating style, you will place yourself in prime position to ascend to the level of that elite, breakaway group regarding health and vitality. It all happens because of your superior metabolic functioning. Any self-imposed physical shackle that held you back in the past—due to eating against nature—will be mitigated, if not totally obliterated. Your days of grappling with metabolic ailments will begin to dissipate. You will feel better and perform at higher levels, with less effort. And the price you must pay is miniscule. All it takes is a little discipline sprinkled throughout your life regarding what you decide to chew on. The result is priceless.

Contrary to what may seem obvious, your boost of energy and augmented quality of life will not be primarily due to the natural foods that you are eating. Believe it or not, that is secondary compared to the new way of thinking you will adopt to engage in a first aisle eating style. It is a decision that will open your eyes wide to greater possibilities throughout the entirety of your life. Essentially you are adopting an elite way of thinking, and this will produce elite results.

The Benefits Are Priceless!

By eating far less processed food, oversaturated with salt, sugar and oil, your taste buds will feel deserted, but eventually they will be reawakened. You will be able to experience a greater variety of gustatory pleasure. Due to eating a higher content of fruits and veggies, your curiosity will be piqued to the cuisine of other cultures and how they spice up their plant-based cuisine. With your increased energy, you will probably want to exercise more, which will push you to eat even better, which will push you to exercise even more—the reciprocal effect is quite profound. On the professional and personal levels, people will be drawn to your enthusiasm and zest for life. The greatest reward is that you will become a beacon of light to colleagues and family who may be quietly battling their own physical ailments. They will notice the changes

> *The most ethical diet just so happens to be the most environmentally sound diet and just so happens to be the healthiest. –* Michael Greger, MD

you have made and become curious about your newfound philosophy. They will wish to emulate you, and you will be in a prime position to help. Lastly, the ripple effect you will have on the ecology and economy is ineffable. You will be consuming fewer and fewer products that harm the environment. Meanwhile, you will be supporting a new economy of health-conscious endeavors that could safeguard the environment. The rewards permeate every aspect of your life, and the rewards are not isolated since there is a societal consequence that has a positive global impact.

Decision Time

Now is the time to leap over the mental and social hurdles of adopting a first aisle eating style. When I first started eating fruits, veggies and grains in 1989, there was not much awareness regarding plant-based eating, but now the road is a lot smoother. Back then most people had never heard the word "vegan." Now more and more restaurants offer vegan options. Although vegan options are a little more available, you must remain inspired and disciplined when you feel yourself succumbing to the guile of highly processed foods and meat products. I admit that it is tough—maybe the toughest endeavor of your life—but it is possible and probable, if you play your cards right.

American culture is firmly entrenched in animal flesh, dairy and processed food. You simply cannot get away from them unless you abandon your family, move to an obscure place, and only then find ground fertile enough to grow your own food. Practically speaking, we know that ain't happenin'. There is a high probability you will stay right here with me in the middle of all the mayhem. Therefore, we must figure out a way to deal with it and enjoy the process.

The first step you must take is to make the decision whether a first aisle eating style makes sense for you in terms of your lifestyle. There is certainly enough proof that it makes sense for you metabolically, but socially it might not seem too appealing. The five stages of REV simply provided a strategy to incorporate a higher percentage of fruits and veggies into your lifestyle. The key to those five stages was that they required minimal discipline because you were not asked to sacrifice any foods you may cherish. Foods you may not have been eating enough of (fresh fruits and veggies) were then injected into your lifestyle. That method is more palatable than giving up foods you love, which can be demoralizing.

Now, you are being asked to sacrifice all meat and dairy products for the greater good. It is a quantum leap and requires much discipline. Yet, if you do so, odds are you will be more energized than ever before. You will have fewer physical ailments. You will age at a slower rate. No credible authority disputes any of that. However, many people do not truly care about any of those benefits, at least not enough to act. Keep in mind REV is not a temporary thing, it is an exciting, lifelong journey. It will never end because you will be enjoying the benefits. The reason you will enjoy the benefits is because you are not sacrificing anything of great value, you are just jettisoning foods that are holding you back. Your decision is an investment in the power of nature with health excellence as your dividend payment.

Second, after deciding to go for it, the process of developing a superior eating style must immediately follow. There are many procrastination techniques I have used to delay my own process of physical vitality. My clients have also contributed techniques of their own. Obviously, all of them are nothing but excuses that we must obliterate.

Nothing but Excuses!

Just in case you may be teetering on the edge regarding whether to dive into a first aisle eating style, following are the excuses I hear all the time. If you are using any of them, it is time to wake up and get a grip on your life.

I'll get started after the holidays. Understand that during the holiday season is when you must be most focused. The only problem is that there is always a holiday around the corner; and let us not forget about birthdays and special occasions. You must get started before the holidays, not after the holidays.

I eat healthy. This is really an indirect excuse born from arrogance. Saying you "eat healthy" usually means you follow all the "scientific" rules and fads of good health. This excuse really says, "I know it all about what to eat."

Unfortunately, that means you are mentally blocked from absorbing anything more than what you think you know. The bottom line is 99% of people who use this excuse are not in the best of shape.

I need protein. This excuse displays complete ignorance of what was put in the Garden of Eden and what composes plants. Protein is in every living thing—including plants—and there is more than enough to sustain a high quality life. And, you can build muscle too!

> *The human body has absolutely no requirement for animal flesh. Nobody has ever been found face-down 20 yards from Burger King because they couldn't get their Whopper in time. – Michael Klaper, MD*

I don't know what to eat. This one is complete denial and disrespect for the plant world. You are just saying you are unwilling to enjoy a simple salad or piece of fruit. Go to your nearest grocery store and hang out in the first aisle for an hour. Then go buy a vegan cookbook. You will figure out what to eat when your belly growls.

It's all genetics. This is a cynical viewpoint and relieves you of responsibility. It assumes one is powerless

> *Nutrition trumps genes. – T. Colin Campbell*

when the power of choice is all we need to make a difference. Your wellbeing is determined by how you allow your genes to be expressed through eating and activity.

I like to eat. This is complete inanity. Doesn't everyone like to eat? (*Actually I know some people who say they don't.*) It assumes enjoyable eating is only possible by consuming what the average American eats. By reading this far you are obviously above average in your desire to try this approach. Putting any and everything in your body is never a sound strategy.

I'm not disciplined. The "woe is me excuse." Give it a break. You are just not incentivized. This type of excuse can change quickly when the doctor gives you the "or else" speech. It is best to "man up" and make a preemptive strike before that happens.

I'll just work it off at the gym. This one is scary because on the surface it makes total sense. The problem is that it gives you license to eat anything because all you must do is sweat enough and the pounds melt away. However, there ain't that much "workin' it off" in the world for most people. It is too time consuming and too stressful on the body. We must "melt it off" through effective eating.

I grew up eating this way. Don't blame your family. I grew up sipping my grandmother's beer! Does that make it the best thing to do? Dangerous eating can become so ingrained in your lifestyle that you disregard what is dangerous. It is senseless and sets you up for failure. We all must mature out of our noxious eating habits and move in a new direction.

I'm too busy to eat healthy. Better eating habits do not take any more time than bad eating habits. All you must do is develop new eating patterns, which will require some discipline. We all have 24 hours, but some of us use that time more wisely than others. It all depends on what is most important to you.

Eating healthy is not convenient. Cheap, fast food is much more convenient because it is cheap and fast—but it is not real food. It is processed and proliferates life-threatening ailments. All you must do is take food with you on your journeys and do not succumb to what is advertised.

It's too expensive to eat healthy. This one seems to be true, but it does not fly, unless you are at the lowest income level. Eating healthier and cheaper than the standard American diet is easier when you cook your own food and shop wisely, especially if you are eating a high percentage of fruit and veggies. There are many great options in the first aisle of the grocery store, as well as the beans and rice aisle, which are less than $1.99 per pound.

My family will not accept it. Whether your family accepts it or not, you must look out for yourself. They will not be able to help you when you are saddled with high blood pressure, high cholesterol or type 2 diabetes, so you must forge your own way. Your family will accept it and cheer you on once you produce positive results.

There's nothing healthy on the menu.
Poppycock! I've heard this one too many times. If so, ask for a special order. Many chefs would love to make something special for you. If not, find a new place to eat.

Everything in Moderation

After breaking through the aforementioned excuses, we must figure out a way to stay on track. We all fall off the path from time to time, but that is just part of the human experience. There is a certain mentality we must be aware of so that we may avoid it. Many will not agree with this, but it is the "everything in moderation" philosophy,

> *Every time sitting at a dining table, we make a choice. Please choose vegetarianism. Do it for the animals. Do it for the environment and for the sake of your own health. — Alec Baldwin*

along with its dastardly cousin, "just a little bit won't hurt." Those two philosophies open the door to all types of undesirable possibilities. Some doors need to be totally shut to move forward unobstructed. Imagine if Alcoholics Anonymous changed its philosophy to "just a little bit of alcohol won't hurt." What if Narcotics Anonymous adopted the "opioids in moderation" policy? It just does not add up, nor does it add up for many other scenarios regarding what you eat.

Look at most people who fall prey to "everything in moderation" or "just a little bit won't hurt." Most lack the discipline to go all the way, so those philosophies are rationalizations to maintain the status quo of their existence. As Michael Greger, MD would say, "Do you want moderate diabetes?" or "Would you like just a little bit of cancer?" Moderate allowances can produce moderate results, or they may produce moderate self-destruction.

Those who believe in those philosophies appear to have a lot of fun, indulging in whatever they care to at any given moment, but the view from the outside is not always clear. I would bet if you spoke with them in a moment of lucidity, many would confess regarding the downside of the "everything in moderation" philosophy in heartbreaking fashion. I once had a friend who broke down and cried after confessing how miserable she was with her weight gain since we left our college days behind us. She was always the life of the party, laughing and drinking the night away. But when the party was over, and we were sitting alone, she broke down and told me how much she was suffering. The "just a little bit" snowflake turned into an avalanche over the course of the last 30 years. Metabolically she was devastated, when just a little discipline would have made all the difference.

The reason those philosophies do not work is because most of us inherently lack the ability to be moderate. "Moderation" is a gray area, whereas total sacrifice of something is black and white. We do better when we commit 100% to one direction.

Eating Out

By reading this far I hope you have decided to go for whole food plant-based eating, 100%, and blast through all procrastination. If so, now the fun begins by facing the social challenges you will surely encounter. Your biggest social challenge: it is 4:59 p.m. and someone comes up with a genius idea to hang out after work for a few drinks. It is a situation where you have little control over where you go. Unless you are with a group of plant-based eaters, odds are you will never go to a health-promoting restaurant where you would be most comfortable. Most likely you will end up at the closest pub with sliders, hot wings and baby-back ribs shoved in your face. Everyone is laughing, drinking and eating everything under the sun. Your resistance begins to wear down. You eat a few pretzels because, "they're only bread." You try a few greasy French fries because, "at least it's potatoes." You are teetering on the brink of complete dietary collapse. Do you cave in?

The best way to deal with situations like that is to fuel up before you go out. Make a pit stop at the nearest place where you can get something plant-based. Usually a convenience store, where you can get fresh fruit and/or nuts, does the trick. When that is not available, sometimes I may try an energy bar. But, beware because most of them are really candy bars. Admittedly, it is not the best option, but when it is the only option, so be it. By fueling up you won't be as tempted to dive into whatever everyone else is eating. Oftentimes, until you get used to a first aisle eating style, you must settle for the lesser of the evils regarding what you eat beforehand.

If you know the establishment you are going to, and you have a little spare time, do the obvious and look at the menu on the Internet. If you do not like what you see, call ahead and ask if you may have something specially prepared for you. Many people are reluctant to do this, as I was at first, but I got over it. You will find most places are willing to accommodate you. Many chefs are tired of cooking the same old thing and are ready, willing and able to take on your request. Remember, chefs are artists and many thrive on creativity. It is your job to give them the inspiration they are craving for. However, oftentimes you are stuck at a place where the food is pre-cooked and microwaved and there is no "chef" to speak of. In those moments, you must make a choice and take what you can get. A salad is not so bad, nor is a hummus vegetable platter!

One of the toughest situations is when you are at a business dinner. Things can get rough. You certainly do not want to make a big commotion and possibly offend clients. You need to make your money like I do; therefore, if possible, exert your influence regarding where you eat and speak with the maître d' ahead of time. If you still have limited options, you may be forced to be content with a poorly concocted salad, soggy vegetables,

> *There is something about veganism that is not easy, but the difficulty is not inherent in veganism, but in our culture.* ~ *Will Tuttle*

bread and pasta. Yes, it sucks, but that's the way it is sometimes. Remember you must keep your clients happy, as well as your body.

Holiday Time

What about Thanksgiving dinner when turkey is the star of the show? Everyone is ready to completely pig out and they are waiting with bated breath to see what you do. You refuse the turkey, ham and all the dairy infused goodies. Then it is time for desert; and you still refrain from partaking. Everyone is staring at you at the dinner table questioning everything you do not eat. Why no turkey? Why no ham? Why no mashed potatoes? Why no macaroni and cheese? Why no stuffing? Why no sweet potato pie? Why no green beans? If you answer any of those questions you spark serious debate. And some people become offended because you appear to be too high and mighty to eat "their food." Most new converts want to avoid the controversy and the easiest way to do that is to just give in and pig out like everyone else. However, as a warning: if you do that, you may start to look and feel like everyone else, usually out of shape and unshapely.

People Think Some Odd Things

Since 1989 I have had many heated family dinner conversations to defend why I converted to a plant-based eating style. If you have had those same conversations, then you will probably notice that many people think and feel in peculiar ways with regard to food and eating habits.

Most people do not pay attention to their health until they are forced to. This is obvious when looking at the stats of obesity and metabolic diseases. The mid-section bulge is particularly dangerous, yet no alarms go off. Then the doctor gives them the "or else" speech about diabetes and heart attacks. Then they will come to see someone in my profession to correct the problem in 30 days. The problem is so much damage could have been done in the previous 30 years that you may not be able to bounce back to optimal health.

Most people don't think about what they eat. We have become so disconnected from plants and animals that we seem to think they originate at the supermarket. Just thinking about the steroids and hormones injected into animals on a farm

> _Recognize meat for what it really is: the antibiotic- and pesticide-laden corpse of a tortured animal. -- Ingrid Newkirk_

makes me nauseous. Maybe it is not obvious, but those steroids and hormones become a part of your physical being once they are digested. It is shocking that so few people in the U.S. are in uproar about it, however, many European countries will not import U.S. meat because of what we pump into our animals.[73] The practices of the food manufacturers have given rise to many documentaries that give us food for thought regarding the horrors of meat and dairy production, such as _Forks Over_

Knives, Food that Kills, and the one receiving much attention in 2017, *What the Health.*

Most people think they're in pretty good physical condition. As a personal trainer, I consider myself an expert when it comes to physical fitness assessments. Maybe I am a tad bit stringent on this topic, but what I see from most people is the complete opposite: poor physical conditioning. An alarming number of people cannot run a mile, cannot do a squat and have no core power. They do not even know that they cannot do those things because they've rarely, if ever, tried to do them. Once they give them a shot, they quickly find out what the real deal is. Unfortunately, believing they're in good physical condition stops them from looking at eating style modifications as a way for improvement.

Most people think doctors have the answers. I love doctors and I have provided personal training for many in the health professions, but this is the scariest of all possibilities. Doctors are masters at prescribing drugs, but not masters at prescribing food. Drugs do not cure metabolic diseases, they simply "manage" them. This is especially evident with maladies like type 2 diabetes and high cholesterol. Most doctors prescribe drugs for those infirmities. However, once you start eating fruits, veggies and grains, cut out meat products and processed food, and begin a serious fitness regimen, those problems start to melt away. Eating and fitness must be your first line of defense. If that does not work, then the drugs will always be there for you.

Most people know nothing about nutrition. Since the 1970s, when fat became demonized, we have been inundated with "food science". There's nothing but mass confusion regarding what nutrients we need. That confusion has created a new market for people looking for "quick fixes" at the supermarket. People want to "buy" health but refuse to eat what will produce the best results. All the while people are getting fatter and sicker, while the answer is in the first aisle of the grocery store.

Stop the Cynicism!

Along with those quirky ways of thinking that can thwart any dietary or fitness program, there is a lot of cynicism regarding a first aisle eating style. Maybe you have heard some of following.

You have to enjoy life! We can all agree on that. The problem with this retort is that it assumes that we all enjoy the same things. Not everyone wants to

> *Veganism is not a sacrifice. It is a joy.*
> *– Gary L. Francione*

drink alcohol to oblivion and gorge on meat, cheese, cake and ice cream. I admit, it is fun to do that, but there are other fun options. Believe it or not, many people thoroughly enjoy fruits, veggies, grains and marvel at what can be created with them.

You're going to die anyway. Assuming that is true, which I hope it is, why is it even being stated? This sentiment gives you license to eat anything and perpetuates a libertine existence. However, to live a higher quality life, some discipline is required. There must be some lines you will not cross, otherwise you run the risk of being run over by metabolic syndrome. It is more fun to spend your life living with zeal rather than suffer with a rotting body, due to an unrestrained existence.

My grandmother smoked, drank whiskey, ate bacon every day and lived to be 100 years old. Yeah, that sounds great, but what type of physical condition was she in? Eating healthier to live longer is secondary to vitality and quality of life. We all know plenty of people who are alive and hanging on at an advanced age, but not truly living. Unfortunately, many are in complete misery. The question is, would grandma have lived a higher quality life if she engaged in a plant-based diet? The answer to that question can never be known, but something tells me she would have.

Humans were designed to eat meat. This statement is just not accurate. It shows complete misunderstanding of the human body. When looking at the anatomy of carnivores versus human beings, it is evident that meat consumption is not the best food for you. You are an herbivore by design. There is no doubt about that. Yes, humans "can" eat meat, but the question is what are our best options? Milton Mills, M.D., does a superb job of answering this question in his YouTube video "Are Humans Designed to Eat Meat?"[74] His analysis tells us that indeed meat is not the solution to a healthier way of life.

Where Do We Go from Here?

As you can see, people believe some odd things. There are lots of excuses being tossed around, as well as myths and facticides, by those who think they "know" the truth. As always, however, the bottom line is positive results. The beauty of our society is that we have freedom of thought and expression, even if those thoughts and expressions are not in our best interest. To go all in and be successful, we must break through self-limiting beliefs perpetuated by those who do not attain positive results.

To make it as easy as possible, forget about all the stats, experiments, surveys and testimonials regarding health and fitness. Most are not accurate, anyway. Odds are, if you want to be wealthy, you would probably listen to a wealthy man. It only makes sense. But, many of us who want to be healthy do not listen to a healthy man. Unwittingly, we listen to those who pitch products, those who are misguided and those who want quick fixes. Most people are following followers, not

> *When a body is in an alkaline state, it avoids disease, but when it's in an acidic state—where you're eating a lot of processed foods, meat, dairy—you're not going to have the hydration in your body, and you're not going to have that ability to fight off disease, and it's going to impact your immune system and the inflammation in your body too. – Vani Hari*

leaders. Therefore, can we ever know what constitutes a "healthy" man or woman? Serious discernment is necessary because far too often we judge who is healthy based on what we see on the surface. What we think is healthy ain't necessarily so.

Countless times I have heard, "Wow, he looked great! He worked out every day, ate healthy and now he has cancer." The outside said one thing, but the inside was in a state of quiet desperation. That said, we must follow a leader; someone whom you respect, someone who yields positive results and is willing to share tips on how he or she got those results.

Did he really eat "healthy"? I know droves of people who get up in the morning, eat their egg whites, a bowl of granola and some yoghurt. The media says this is a "healthy" meal, you get plenty of protein and you are off to a running start. Ninety-nine percent of people would agree, but not me. Although, on the outside, many people who adhere to that way of starting the day may look great. But, we do not know what will happen in the long term. I predict something undesirable because all that is being consumed is what the advertisers and salesmen say should be consumed. Unfortunately, their ways of thinking are often biased for the sake of financial gain, and many of us tacitly allow ourselves to be subject to their views; suffering then manifests and few of us complain. So, where do we go from here?

The 1st Aisle is as much about faith as it is about empirical evidence or scientific proof. Sometimes there is just no way to know, but faith mixed with common sense has been the guiding light for many. Observe people, take note of what they do and follow the person who is the archetype of what you value most. Regarding health and fitness, I say look at the woman or man you can find with the most energy; best physique; best disposition about life; and one who performs at the highest level possible. That is the person to take counsel from. Whether you have personal or even tangential experience with that individual, he or she is the one to follow when it comes to staying young and living healthy. You must have faith that you are making the right decision based on all the information you have gathered and studied. My studies and experience have led me to understand that whole food plant-based eating is the best way to go. You will most likely come to the same conclusion the deeper you dig for information and the more you experiment.

> *Every year, the average American eats as much as 33 pounds of cheese. That's up to 60,000 calories and 3,100 grams of saturated fat. So why do we eat so much cheese? Mainly it's because the government is in cahoots with the processed food industry. And instead of responding in earnest to the health crisis, they've spent the past 30 years getting people to eat more. This is the story of how we ended up doing just that. –Michael Moss*

If you decide to go with a first aisle eating style, you will be pleased to find that it is a growing movement which will expand your belief system. More people are becoming more conscious of how eating determines overall health and wellness. More people are looking at the man in the mirror to take responsibility for health instead of putting total faith in the medical professions. And personal responsibility will rise even further as health care costs continue to escalate and very few people are being healed.

Finally, is there a metabolic downside by converting to a first aisle eating style? Absolutely not! But, most of the public has not considered

> *Let food be thy medicine and medicine be thy food. -*
> *- Hippocrates*

it due to lack of education, marketing and experience. Once your body begins to respond positively, you will know there is an easy answer to your health woes. It is hard to deny the obvious when your weight stabilizes, you get sick less often and you feel like moving around to burn off energy. Believe it or not, you really do feel much younger. However, do not be in a rush for excellence. Oftentimes, it may take a while to dig out of a hole. Unbeknownst to you, your body may have been used and abused for quite some time. Give it the time to turn in the right direction and do not look back.

Go all in and hang out in the first aisle!

CALL TO ACTION

Objective: *Be an inspiration to others by exhibiting health, happiness and youth through the power of The 1st Aisle.*

Although man has included meat in his diet for thousands of years, his anatomy and physiology, and the chemistry of his digestive juices, are still unmistakably those of a frugivorous animal.

Herbert M. Shelton

Appendix A - My Day as a 1st Aisler

1st Aisler: A person who overcomes the negative effects of preservatives, additives, processing aids and other chemicals found in processed food through eating fresh produce from the first aisle of the grocery store. The 1st Aisler strives for the following:

1. Eats fresh produce from the first aisle of the grocery store. (Exceptions are aisles where there are grains, beans, nuts and water.)
2. Prepares hand-made meals at home or in a kitchen, striving to avoid oils, condiments or any mass manufactured products.
3. Eats organically grown produce, depending on availability and price.
4. Meals eaten outside of the home are restricted to as few as possible (0-20%) or as little as lifestyle will allow.
5. Meals eaten outside of the home are vegan.

Vegan: A person who eats plant-based foods, including vegetables, fruits, legumes, seeds, beans, nuts and whole grains, including processed foods made from plants. Anything made with animals is not permitted, such as leather, wool, gelatin, beeswax, or lanolin.

Whole Food Plant-Based: A person who eats plant-based foods like a vegan, but excludes processed food, such as oil, white flour, and refined sugar. It is based on unprocessed or minimally processed veggies, fruits, whole grains, beans, legumes, nuts, and seeds.

Most people are astonished that I have not "intentionally" eaten animal products over the last 30 years. However, there have been numerous times that I did not know what I was eating when someone said the food was "vegetarian." For instance, I've gone to restaurants where the waiter swore the soup had no animal products in it, only to find out on a subsequent visit that it was made with chicken stock. Recently I found that a vegetarian sushi roll I routinely order from a Japanese restaurant contained fish eggs (masago). Another time I found that eggs were added to a veggie stir fry I fancied. Of course, I'm dismayed when I learn these things because those foods are now banished to my "do not chew" list. Since those types of scenarios have popped up over the last 30 years, I no longer refer to myself as "vegan."

My goal is to eat as much food as possible from the first aisle of the grocery store. This is especially true of raw vegetation that would be tons of fruits and salads. Beyond that, when I eat out of my home and venture into the unknown, I order food which I believe is plant-based, although I'm sure lots of it is rife with chemicals because processed food is used by most cooks (e.g., sauces, condiments, any packaged product). The only way to be totally pure regarding the best food to eat is to grow your own food and cook it yourself—what a social nightmare that would be. I'd never go out on a date! So, I now refer to myself as a "First Aisler" regarding my eating style. I'm basically a person who strives for a whole food plant-based existence. I eat veggies, fruits and grains, with minimal to no processing.

There is much danger when eating beyond that first aisle. For most Americans, each day is rife with processed food consumption because we do not think about it. Its potential effects do not scare us enough to take measures against it immediately, partly because the effects are long term and we cannot feel immediate pain. If we do not get sick immediately—and receive maximum pleasure from what is swirling around in our mouths—it is easy to overlook food indiscretions. For instance, to make French fries only two ingredients are necessary: potatoes and oil. Yet McDonald's French Fries produced in the United States contain 14 ingredients.[75] European McDonald's French Fries contain only four ingredients.[76,77] Could those 10 extra ingredients—possibly toxic and banned in Europe, but not in the U.S.—cause us unintended harm? Many would say the 10 extra chemicals are innocuous, but I would disagree. Therefore, my number one priority is to avoid as many toxic ingredients in food as possible. The best way to do that would be to sell all my worldly possessions, scour the world for fertile ground, grow my own crops and don't worry, be happy. Admittedly, I'm too much of a scaredy-cat to do that. The second-best option is to be a First Aisler. That we can all do.

"Where do you get your protein from?" is a question I'm frequently asked. That question is often followed by, "What do you eat?" My routine is simple during working days, Monday thru Saturday. Since my working hours are sporadic, I am not in a 9 to 5 routine. Normally I arise between 5am to 6am for early morning training appointments. The first thing I do is drink a quart of water, which I do 95% of the time before eating anything for the day. The 5% of the time that I do not drink my quart of water is when I may not have access to a men's room for the next few hours (e.g., long car or train rides). Also, I normally do not eat anything the first hour or so after I wake up. A quart of water really fills you up and I am not immediately hungry. Then, after a training session or two, I usually eat bananas, maybe two or three. I'm a banana fiend because they are so easy to work with. No rinsing necessary, just peeling. Also, they are not juicy, so you do not have to be concerned about your hands getting wet. Sometimes I'll have oranges or apples, depending on what is accessible and appealing. Suffice it to say, before noon I easily consume at least five pieces of fruit.

Often I eat salad for breakfast. I may have back-to-back training sessions at 6 and 7 a.m., with a one-hour break at 8 a.m. I have the luxury of living within two minutes of where I work, so I can run home, eat a salad, and be back for a 9 a.m. training session. I prefer salad for breakfast, the only drawback is the time it takes to prepare it. Needless to say, I am rushing around in the morning like everyone else.

Around lunchtime I normally have another salad. I truly believe that salad is the key to a successful existence, so my philosophy is to eat as much as possible. Six out of seven days a week, I eat a minimum of two large salads.

Oftentimes I will eat three or four, if I do not eat cooked food for the day. Why so much salad? It's all about fiber! My belief is that fiber carries toxicity out of your body, so it's the antidote to all the processed food we consume. Plus, I love the taste of it! Regarding contents, my favorite salad is spinach, radicchio, field greens, apple, avocado, and jalapeno peppers with squeezed lime juice and/or apple cider vinegar. This salad I make myself with ingredients from the first aisle of the grocery store. In years past I would go to salad bars almost every day, typically at Whole Foods. My salad would weigh a minimum of 1.75 pounds, oftentimes tumbling over two pounds, at a cost of $16 to $18. I would fill it with uncooked and cooked vegetation, but I rarely do that nowadays. There are all types of oils, salts and possibly nauseous bacteria that could be lurking in the prepared foods of salad bar, so I tread lightly in that area. My only pitfall is that I may pick up a few roasted Brussel sprouts or cauliflower florets to munch on as I'm shopping. (*Oops—hope I don't get arrested!*)

Dinnertime is usually sautéed veggies (no oil, just water) with quinoa, rice or baked potatoes, with avocado added and lime juice. My favorite ingredients are mixed into a huge pot, including broccoli, carrots, kale, onions, garlic and jalapeno peppers. Sometimes I'll add in fresh dill, parsley or cilantro. Depending on how I'm feeling, I may mix in some ingredients like squash, cauliflower or apples. I'm not a chef by any means and this is what I cook 99% of the time. Having sautéed veggies daily does not bother me a bit, but I'm sure most people would get bored. I believe there are more than enough veggies for me to swap in and out, so I'm always entertained with my dinner. As with breakfast and lunch, I'm striving for high fiber content, as well as gustatory pleasure.

As the day progresses, I eat more fruit, but a problem for me is that I sometimes eat too much late at night. For instance, I may eat two or three bananas before going to bed, along with a couple of mangos. They're like candy to me, but I sometimes get a tummy ache! Or, I may eat a huge salad before going to bed after late training appointments. Those late-night activities I do not advise at all, but who among us is perfect? By the end of the day I have usually eat ten pieces of fruit or more. The few times this does not happen is when I'm on vacation or working crazy hours and forget to eat.

For breakfast, lunch and dinner, the goal is to avoid all added processing aids, preservatives, artificial flavorings and chemicals. Nothing I use is packaged in any form. No salt or seasonings from a shaker, oil from a bottle or anything canned, except for rice, millet, farro, quinoa or other grains that may be packaged. Another exception is ground flaxseed, which provides an oily consistency if I do not have avocado. (*By the way, I eat lots of avocado, at least three per day.*) They're oily and I cannot get enough of them. The first thing people bellow when they find that out is, "It's so fattening!" My response, "So what." If it is "so fattening" it is unprocessed fat, which is certainly not a problem. Aside from that, there is hardly any fat in my daily diet, so I never think about fat content in my food.

The amount of fiber that I consume may sound extreme, but, as aforementioned, it is my armor against all the toxicity I may consume when I eat out. For instance, you go to a friend's barbeque and you eat the corn salad, which you are told is all vegetables. You partake of it and it tastes great, but I'd bet my last dollar the dressing put on it came from a bottle with added preservatives and chemicals. Eating at restaurant is precarious also. I enjoy Thai food, but are my veggies most likely cooked on the same grill as meats, chemicals and who knows what else. I do not care enough to interrogate the sous chef, so I have no idea what is going on. It's dangerous out there! But if it really bothers you that much, your best bet is to stay home and rattle your own pots and pans. Again, my defense and antidote against added toxicity is tons of fiber from the first aisle.

When I eat out of my home I write down everything that I eat. My goal is to go two consecutive days only eating the food I prepare at home. It may sound easy, but it is very difficult to do when you grow up in a culture rife with processed food. When I am not in the mood to cook my own veggies, sometimes I may order steamed veggies from my favorite Chinese restaurant, then add my own spices, peppers, avocado and lemon/lime juice. *(By the way, Asian restaurants are the greatest because they always seem to have a steamed veggie selection on the menu!)* Sometimes I order veggie primavera with gluten free pasta from my favorite Italian restaurant. I'm not too sure if I'm allergic to gluten, but I feel as though it inflames my sinuses. If I eat too much regular pasta during the evening, I find it difficult to breathe and fall asleep at night. Also, it bloats my belly. When I visit my family in Texas we may go to stir fry restaurants and exotic salad bars. There's a new vegan diner my little sister discovered, and I love it. It's pure vegan junk food! *(Be careful with food labeled "vegan," most of it is still junk.)* Sometimes I drive into Manhattan and go to my favorite vegan spots, something I used to do at least twice a week in years past. The few times I eat anything with added sugar is when I go to vegan restaurants and order chocolate cake or pie. It's amazing what you can do without eggs and dairy. Sometimes I'll go out for a mixed drink. Vodka and grapefruit *(affectionately known as a Greyhound)* is my favorite. I also love a nice glass of scotch, especially after a round of golf or after dinner. I receive gift bottles during the holidays. Rarely do I drink beer because it causes the dreaded beer belly. All those things I write down. If I get sick I am able to trace my eating activity and hopefully identify any problem

All the aforementioned I enjoy immensely, but I still consider those indulgences dangerous and poisonous, so they must be limited. My saving grace is, as much as I enjoy them, I enjoy eating from the first aisle just as much, because it gives me the results I desire. I pray that the fiber is escorting the toxicity from my body every day. It took me way too long—more than 50 years—to understand that the first aisle has the answers I had been looking for, but now I got it. My best advice: become a First Aisler and don't look back.

Appendix B – The Age of the Resultatarian®

Resultatarian® Tenets

1. *The universe is wiser than man.* Whatever entity brought us into existence is omniscient and omnipotent. Whether you refer to it as nature, god, the universe or something else, it understands the innerworkings of the human body far more than humans do. Oftentimes we tend to believe that the discoveries of man are more powerful than the creations of the universe, as we rely on those with advance degrees for advice. But, whatever they know pales in comparison to all there is to know. What is natural always has the upper hand compared to what man creates.

2. *Long-term results are more important than short-term results.* Many results bring us immediate and momentary pleasure, but those results dissipate because they were designed to be long term. Visualize the far-reaching outcome of your actions to make the best decisions in the moment, which guarantee long-term results. Oftentimes immediate results are not discernible as they lay the foundation for long-term results. Patience is the key to lifelong sustainability and joy.

3. *The 1st aisle is your first defense.* Since the universe has put all the nutrients we need in the soil, plant life must be treasured as nature's conduit. Your body is under constant attack by viruses, bacteria, air pollution, mental stress, physical trauma and the toxic food we eat. Eating as much plant-based food as possible is your best defense. If you cannot get your plants

directly from the farm, the first aisle is there to serve you. It's your first defense and your best defense.

The tenets of Resultatarianism are intended to be a guide to produce desired results through plant-based eating, not as dogma or doctrine. The objective is to be in accord with the infinite wisdom of nature. When we are successful, we wear protective armor against bacteria, viruses, allergies, as well as metabolic diseases. When we fight against nature, by refusing to eat plants, we open a Pandora's box of stress and disease.

Frustration can set in when results are not easily discernible. Often what we are searching for is not detectable by the naked eye; therefore, patience must be invoked as the process of success takes root. Feel and faith must guide you through the initial stages of results, which is ongoing and increases in momentum as time goes on. There are three ways of measuring results from a Resultatarian perspective:

1. **Weight Control.** Most people want to hit a specific number on the scale, which is understandable. It is easy to "see" the number and we have become accustomed to the bathroom scale being in control. If you are a six feet tall male, 60 years old, the height/weight ratio stats say a safe weight is 160 to 196 pounds. However, that is not how I measure weight, which, ironically, I do not

believe should be a concern at all. For the Resultatarian the telltale sign regarding weight is midsection girth. A protruding belly is clearly an issue. If you can grab more than an inch, there

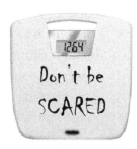

is an issue to address. If you can grab a handful or more of adipose tissue, serious and immediate intervention is needed. On the opposite end of the spectrum, it would be great to see some muscle striations. The coveted abdominal 6-pack is perfect! If you lift your shirt and you see definition, odds are your weight is perfect, regardless of what the scale says.

2. **Energy Level.** This one is tricky because most of my clients think I am overzealous when it comes to energy. At this point I am of the

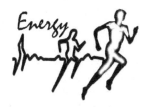

philosophy that I should have the energy level of someone two-thirds my age. As of this writing, I'm 54 years old, therefore I should have the energy level of a male 36 years old. Of course, that could be achieved through various pharmaceuticals that are not in the first aisle, but that is not what the tenets of Resultatarianism are based on. The most efficient way for me to achieve that result is through eating plant-based foods, while eschewing processed food, alcohol, OTC drugs, and NSAIDS (non-steroidal anti-inflammatory drugs) as much as possible. When it is done the natural food way, your body will have greater power over an extended period of time. Perhaps until the day you die!

3. **Toxicity Control.** If your body was a garbage can and it began to fill up, eventually it must be emptied. But, what if it was not emptied and it began to overflow? The stench would be noxious, it would become an eyesore to 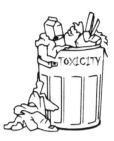 the community and a hazard to your neighbors. Too often we fill out bodies with toxicity and it overflows, therefore it must be emptied, which is the process of "catching a cold" to release the toxicity. Other forms of toxicity release could be through skin rashes, headaches, fevers, cramping, nausea or whatever else derails you and forces you to take a timeout. Therefore, the first objective is to slow down the rate at which we fill the body with toxicity. The second objective is to empty the toxicity before it gets anywhere near full. If we accomplish those two goals, we will get sick far less

often and much less virulently. Hence, maybe we will sneeze instead of cough. Maybe we will feel tired instead of getting a fever. Maybe we will only feel sick every six months instead of every month. And, just maybe we can live a minimally toxic life until the day we die.

Oftentimes the desire for immediate physical results overpowers reason and sensibility. For instance, high protein/low carb diets (or ketogenic diets), such as the Atkins Diet or South Beach Diet, defies reason because it is a diet that you cannot engage in for the entirety of your life, without detrimental effects. Additionally, in the short term it can be dangerous because you trick your body into believing it is starving and you slip into ketosis to burn more fat instead of carbohydrates. I have known many who have successfully lost weight on the Atkins Diet in the short term, but they all gained it back after reverting to their traditional diets. Their goal was usually to lose weight for some imminent event, such as a wedding or summer vacation. During the process some developed kidney stones because of the high protein philosophy of the diet and had to be hospitalized. Others became ill due to their bodies being in a highly acidic state.

Assuming Dr. Atkins followed his own diet, he did not appear to be the picture of health when he died in 2003, due to complications of a slip and fall accident where he injured his head. Prior to the accident, he went into cardiac arrest in 2002. Subsequent to his death, it has been reported that he showed signs of heart disease on his autopsy report—claims disputed by his family and private doctors—so his health and diet had been heavily scrutinized over his lifetime and beyond.[78] Short term the Atkin's Diet works like a charm, long term it appears to fail, so why do it? The ketogenic diets surely do not adhere to the tenets of Resultatarianism.

My clients understandably want to see improvement over the short term, but I am always looking long term, usually twenty years into the future. One objective of **The 1st Aisle** and Resultatarianism is to make you feel and look better immediately; but, as importantly, to weed out problems before they take root and possibly cripple your future. The only way to achieve those objectives is by looking long term. Unfortunately, we have all known those who are debilitated or have lost their lives due to not taking the long germ seriously. To prevent that we must focus on producing maximum results through marrying the lifestyle you want to live (short term goals) with what is in your best interest (long term goals). It is a balancing act that we must embrace to bring lifelong joy and well-being.

Appendix C – What is Processed Food?

There has been much controversy regarding what constitutes processed food. I consider *anything eaten that has lost the human touch* to be processed food. It is food usually prepared by machines in a factory (not cooked by human hands); it is food mass manufactured using chemicals, processing aids and additives (unnatural non-food products); and it is food packaged for sale using preservatives (for added shelf life and transportation), all of which is done to maximize profitability. In a nutshell, processed food is something you would never cook in your kitchen. However, I have had much verbal jousting with those who are nitpicky and say, if you slice an apple with a knife, then that is processing. Technically speaking they are correct, but if I slice an apple in my kitchen by hand, I do not see any harm in that.

Maybe we should be aware of what the major food manufacturing companies think of as processed food. Joanna Blythman, author of *Swallow This: Serving Up the Food Industry's Darkets Secrets*, gives explicit detail regarding the inner workings of the processed food industry. Although much of her research was based in Europe, the food processing companies are international conglomerates using the same methods worldwide. Robert Lustig, M.D., references *Swallow This* in his YouTube video "Processed Food: An Experiment That Failed" and he details the objectives of the processed food manufacturers. Their mission is to make processed food a commodity (storable food), so it will not spoil easily or quickly, thereby increasing its economic value.[79] To achieve that objective—basically commoditizing the product—

processed food has certain qualities from a *food engineering perspective*:

1. Must be able to be mass-produced.
2. Must be consistent batch to batch.
3. Must be consistent country to country.
4. Contains specialized ingredients from specialized companies (trade secrets).
5. Virtually all macro-nutrients are frozen (therefore fiber must be removed).
6. Must stay emulsified (water and fat don't separate) and food product must not fall apart.
7. Must have long shelf-life or freezer life for transportation purposes.

The processed foods that those companies produce are mainly found in the center aisles of the grocery store. Compared to what is in the first aisle of the grocery store, those foods can be dangerous to your health over the long term. You certainly cannot base your diet on them and expect superior health results. They should be regarded as treats, if consumed at all, after you have eaten predominantly from the first aisle.

From a *nutrition perspective*, processed food is defined by little to no:[80]

1. Fiber: necessary for optimal digestion. Gut bacteria feed from fiber.
2. Omega-3 fatty acids.

3. Micronutrients/Phytochemicals: vitamins and minerals necessary for optimal metabolic functioning.

And it is also defined by too much:

1. Trans fats: man made fat which bacteria does not digest so food does not become rancid. Trans fats are becoming extinct in the American food supply.
2. Additives: used for flavoring, coloring, etc. Many are known to be toxic.
3. Salt: could cause high blood pressure.
4. Nitrates: preservatives and fertilizers that cause cell damage.
5. Sugar: sweeteners that cover up bad tastes.
6. Branch Chain Amino Acids (BCAs: leucine, isoleucine, valine): they build muscle and could be turned into liver fat in excess. Corn fed meat has this, grass fed meat not as much.
7. Omega-6 Fatty Acids: lead to arachidonic acid and prostaglandins, which are inflammatory mediators.
8. Emulsifiers: detergents that deteriorate the mucin layer in the intestines, leading to leaky gut (polysorbate-80, carboxymethylcellulose, carrageenan). Could be associated with autoimmune diseases and allergies.

From a *human experience perspective*, Joanna Blythman lists the defining characteristics of processed food and gives explicit detail regarding each characteristic:[81]

1. Sweet
2. Salty
3. Oily
4. Flavored
5. Colored
6. Watery
7. Starchy
8. Tricky (clean food labeling)
9. Old (shelf-life extension)
10. Packed (packaging)

To produce those characteristics the processed food industry uses some of the various types of agents and/or additives: emulsifiers, stabilizers, sequestrants (meat binders), gelling agents, thickeners, anti-foaming agents, bulking agents, carriers, carrier solvents, emulsifying salts, firming agents, flavor enhancers, flour-treatment agents, foaming agents, glazing agents, humectants, desiccants, propellants, raising agents, flavor carriers and binders. In excessive amounts, all the aforementioned could be toxic to the human body, hence processed food is considered by many to be extremely dangerous.

Aside from what we know is in processed food through labeling, there are also things that are not required to be on a food label. Processing aids (a subcategory of "incidental additives") are substances that are approved by both the Food and Drug Administration (FDA) and the U.S. Department of Agriculture (USDA). They are not substances that you would eat as a food in any way, but they are used in the production of all types of foods. Supposedly they are not present in significant amounts once the food becomes a finished product. Processing aids are not required to be on food labels if they meet one of the following criteria:[82]

1. It's added to the food but later removed.

2. It's added to the food, but gets converted into a substance already present in the food.

3. It's added for a technical effect during processing but isn't present at "significant" levels in the food.

Although the USDA and FDA consider processing aids as products generally regarded as safe (GRAS), the government and food industry have been wrong in the past. We are now all aware of the fiasco with margarine and trans fats. As of now, we have no idea how dangerous these products could be.

The American public consumes all types of foods that use processing aids with reckless abandon. For instance, many enzymes are considered to be processing aids, which are used as catalysts to speed up chemical reactions. In nature they are proteins that occur naturally in the cells of plants, animals and microorganisms. In commercial terms enzymes are used for industrial applications to make items such as laundry detergents, contact lens cleaners and chemicals to stone wash jeans. There are thousands of other applications that use these very toxic substances. If you swallow them, an immediate trip to the emergency room must follow. Sad to say that that those same chemicals are used in food production to maximize profit, yet do not have to be put on the food contents label. Are food-processing enzymes truly safe over the long term? It's anyone's guess.

Usually enzymes end with "ase", such as:[83]

1. Amylase used in brewing.
2. Invertase used to keep food soft and chewy.
3. Amyloglucosidase used to give bread an even, brown crust.
4. Maltogenic amylase used to slow the rate at which food stales.
5. Pectin methylesterase used to keep frozen fruits and veggies firmer.
6. Lipases used to create cheese flavors.
7. Pectinase used to make juice clear rather than cloudy and to firm up fruit so it retains its shape during processing.

There are 10 companies that control 90% all the processed food in the world.[84] Whenever you consume anything that is bottled, wrapped, boxed or canned, you know who to thank:

1. Nestlé
2. PepsiCo
3. Unilever
4. Coca-Cola

5. Mars
6. Mondelez
7. Danone
8. General Mills
9. Associated British Foods
10. Kellogg's

Appendix D – The Importance of Exercise

The importance of exercise for your well-being must not be underestimated. Its benefits include enhanced strength and functionality, pain relief, and injury prevention. And, let's face it, we all want to look strong, svelte and sexy. However, we must be clear that physical exercise does not outweigh the power of plant-based eating regarding your "metabolic" strength. There are many people who exercise feverishly, on a daily basis, and still do not get the results they greatly desire. They believe they can "work the weight off" and overcome chronic disease through an accelerated heart rate and pouring sweat, but that philosophy is ill-fated. Yes, exercise is critical, but it does not get you across the finish line. Instead, we must "melt the weight off" and overcome disease through consuming the appropriate healing foods, which are plant-based. Then we can use exercise and reap all its benefits.

There are six types of exercise I recommend for my clients:

1. Cardio (running, jogging, elliptical)
2. Core (sit-ups, planks, squats, body weight exercises)
3. Flexibility (stretching, yoga)
4. Resistance (weights, weight machines)
5. Plyometrics (sprinting, jumping, explosive movements)
6. Corrective (healing injury or chronic pain)

Of the six types of exercise, I am of the belief that cardio, core and flexibility are essential to engage in, on a consistent basis. If they are neglected, you will pay a heavy price regarding movement and functionality as you age.

The comfort and enjoyment you may have, in all activities, could be totally disrupted.

In American culture the heart needs more stimulation than the average person's daily regimen gives it. Many of us sit down all day at work, which is so detrimental that sitting is being compared to smoking.[85] The best way to counter the negative effects of sitting is with cardio exercise. Jogging is my favorite and I frequently run three to five miles. Most people find it difficult to jog around the block or walk up a flight of stairs. The heart starts pounding, breathing becomes arduous and a total collapse is imminent. This must change to make progress physically and bolster your cardiovascular system.

Next core work is critical because is strengthens the spine and supports all body movements. Your first exercise of the day is a core exercise, usually a sit-up, which you do when sitting up from your bed. Then most people stand up from a sitting position, performing the ascending movement of a squat. That movement utilizes your back, abs, glutes and other supporting muscles. It may surprise you to know how many people find it difficult to perform those two basic tasks. Your core is working all day long, but for the average person it only gets the minimal amount of work it needs, via daily tasks. Since many of us do not perform strenuous tasks during the day, the core suffers. Hence, more than 31 million Americans suffer from back pain and it is the second leading cause of visits to the doctor (second to upper-respiratory infections).[86]

Flexibility exercises are extremely important, but often neglected. From my experience people who work out the most do the least of it, in proportion to how much they exercise. When you work out on a consistent basis your muscles, tendons and ligaments become tight and more susceptible to injury. Therefore, flexibility exercises are recommended before and after exercise. They are akin to putting oil in an engine. Stretching and yoga I strongly recommend. When you incorporate them all movements are much easier and smoother.

Resistance training (weight lifting) I do not consider to be critical. Your natural body weight can provide more than enough resistance. However, lifting weights will certainly help, as it builds stronger muscles, bones, tendons and ligaments. It will help with your other workouts also, but be careful of going overboard with it. When most men think of working out they think about pumping iron. They immediately jump into chest and arm exercises and neglect the rest of the body. But, most people who are musclebound tend to be very inflexible and find it difficult to perform movements that require dexterity, agility and finesse.

Plyometric training is fun and requires much energy, but it is difficult for most. I do this the least with my clients because many of them are middle-aged and their joints may not be strong enough for jumping, sprinting and other explosive movements. Many people come to me with knee, hip and lower back pain, which would only be exacerbated by plyometric exercises. But, for those who can handle plyometrics, go for it and have some fun. They are the most exhilarating of the types of exercises. However, before you start doing them, play it safe and be sure to engage in plenty of cardio, flexibility and core exercises.

Corrective exercises I use when clients have had injuries or chronic pain. Many have been through physical therapy sessions, but insurance will not pay for it any longer. That is when personal training is the next likely option. These exercises are usually simpler because the individual's primary concern may be healing compared to muscle building, functionality and beautification.

Producing the energy necessary to exercise is of prime importance. Your body burns three types of fuel to produce ATP (adenosine triphosphate), referred to as the chemical energy of life: creatine phosphate, glycogen and adipose fatty acids. ATP directly powers myosin, the protein immediately responsible for converting chemical energy into movement. All muscle cells contain stored ATP, but only in minimal amounts, so producing ATP is a critical function of your metabolism. The first energy production source used is the conversion of creatine phosphate into ATP, but it only gives you enough energy for about 5 to 10 seconds. The next energy source to be used is glycogen, which is stored in your muscles and liver. This is your body's preferred fuel for energy, but it takes longer than creatine phosphate to be converted to ATP. If it's not replenished during exercise, glycogen usually lasts from 20 to 90 minutes, depending on the intensity of exercise. Last, fat is used for energy, but the process of converting fat to energy may take 30 minutes or so to kick in. It is the most abundant and concentrated source of energy the body has.[87]

Due to the different energy sources utilized by the body, it's wise to engage in all the forms of exercise. I know plenty of people who do only one type of exercise that they are great at, but they are still not in the best physical condition. For instance, there's a big difference between sprinting and jogging, although both are running. Those two activities utilize the same muscles but have significantly different impacts on your metabolism, musculature and cardiovascular system. I enjoy both and would recommend engaging in both. If you are a high performance, competitive athlete, of course you would specialize in one area, but cross training is highly recommended for the average person. It gives you the balance you need to look and feel great.

For my clients I usually recommend 40 minutes of cardio exercise, three times a week. I believe cardio is the most important type of exercise and it does not matter what the activity is: jogging, biking, elliptical, walking, dancing, etcetera. The key to cardio is to enjoy it. In our face-paced world we want everything to be expedient so we can move onto the next task, but cardio can be slow and laborious. Therefore, do what you must to make it enjoyable. Join an exercise group, take classes, use your ear buds with your favorite music; basically do whatever it takes. You must build your VO2 max (maximal oxygen uptake), which is the rate at which your body can process oxygen, and exercise your slow twitch muscles (glutes, hamstrings, calves, quads) to strengthen your cardio vascular system and promote endurance. Given rates of cardiovascular disease in this country, in the long run your heart will thank you for it.

My recommendation for core exercise is at least twice per week for about 30 minutes. I tell all my clients, "It's a butt and gut world." When the gut and the butt are strong, everything else falls into place. The core supports all movement and must be exercised through sit-ups, planks, squats, etcetera. One of the issues we must grapple with over time is the power of gravity. As we get older we slump over more because gravity is pulling us down to the ground and our muscles are not as powerful to keep us upright. Hence, we have postural issues and movement becomes more difficult. Pain can radiate from the lower back, which can have a ripple effect throughout the rest of the body. By simply doing core exercises you will alleviate back and hip pain, have greater functionality and feel much better. You may even develop the coveted six-pack abs.

One area where most of us stumble is flexibility exercise. Most people I know who work out above and beyond the call of duty do not stretch anywhere near enough. They feel tight and achy and are more susceptible to injury, therefore I recommend stretching every day for at least 15 minutes. Pay special attention to stretching the back, hips and hamstrings. Those areas appear to cause the most amount of problems. To the dismay of my yoga colleagues, I view yoga and stretching as basically the same, except yoga requires more strength and stamina. That said, I strongly advise yoga classes. Yoga can build tremendous core stamina and balance, while at the same time stretching the muscles and tendons.

One of the excuses we concoct for not getting enough of the essential exercises is lack of time, therefore in 2012 I authored a book, **The 2-Minute Office Workout** (http://corecommando.com/2-minute-office-workout/). It covers many exercises and stretches you can perform in the comfort of your working environment, without breaking a sweat. If you do nothing else, at the very least take a timeout for two minutes every hour and try the exercises and stretches. It does not take much to keep your muscles activated like an oiled engine, but it does take consistency. There are three exercises that I believe must be mastered to maintain functionality as we get older: squats, planks and tummy crunches. Examples of those exercises are on the previously mentioned website.

Appendix E – Kickstart Your Metabolism

Sometimes you need to tweak your daily regimen to induce a metabolic kickstart. Making lifestyle changes is always a tough proposition, so small, bite-sized chunks are most effective for people on the run. Many people want to "boost" or "rev up" their metabolism through exotic drinks and excessive exercise so it burns more fat. That philosophy has become very popular these days because it gives you the option to maintain some of your ill-fated eating habits. Needless to say, that method is not getting the job done for most Americans. As you age your metabolism may slow down, but I'm of the opinion that the deceleration of one's metabolism is mainly due to overtaxing the body with the chemicals and toxins found in processed food. Food additives, processing aids, preservatives, adulterants, etcetera, make your blood more acidic and invoke immune system responses that hamper the digestive system. When those chemicals are consumed year after year, your metabolism is thrown off track and all hell breaks loose.

The remedy is not to "boost" or "rev up" your metabolism, but to "optimize" it so it works in your favor. It's at its best when it efficiently burns fuel, eliminates toxins and strengthens your immune system, which is heavily influenced by what you eat. Many people find it exceptionally difficult to "optimize" their metabolism because it may involve multiple steps. *The 1st Aisle* contains only six steps, but for those who find it too daunting, I offer metabolic kick-starters to get the ball rolling.

The following kick-starters are not in sequential order. I suggest only trying one or maximum two at a time for at least two weeks. Undoubtedly the one you pick will open the door to better food choices and give you time to reflect on your overall lifestyle.

1. **Prepare your own food.** The greatest disconnect we have from the rest of the world is that we outsource cooking. It is easier to have someone else cook for us and we have the cash to pay for it. Americans probably eat out more than any other nation because we have access to so much. I have a dear friend, Anni Monkkonen from Jyväskylä, Finland who said that before coming to America her family only "ate out" once per week. As soon as she came over to America her family wanted to try all the varieties of food we have. Everything was so sugary and delicious. She even brought some bread for me from Finland to show the difference in sweetness. Immediately they all started gaining weight. Preparing your own food, regardless of what or how you eat, gives you control and instills discipline regarding your eating choices.

2. **Eat a "huge" salad every day.** Maybe you remember the "big salad" episode of Seinfeld of years ago. If so, eat a salad twice as big each day. Fiber is the magic ingredient for supreme digestion, but meat products and process food contain little to none of it. Every day, mostly twice a day, I eat a huge salad with spinach, field greens, avocado,

apple and onion. I chop up some jalapeno pepper to give it a little kick, then I squeeze fresh lime juice on it. Give that a shot, but feel free to use any "natural" ingredient in it that you get from the first aisle of the grocery store. Nothing from a bottle or can, with only plant fare in it. Your digestive system will be very pleased once you give it a daily shot of fiber.

3. **The 3-to-1 Plan.** Every time you eat something you believe is unhealthy, like a dinner consisting of cheeseburgers and fries, you must eat three huge salads and 5 pieces of fruit to counter it. Or, you could determine the caloric content of the cheeseburger and fries and eat the same number of calories as a salad and fruit. Raw fruits and veggies will help you neutralize the devastating effects of junk food.

4. **Keep all processed sweets out of the home.** This is very difficult to do for those who have a "sweet tooth," but if it's not in front of you, you will not desire it as much. Processed sugar is an addictive drug, so let your sweet tooth be satisfied with fruit. You will be amazed by how sweet and satisfied it is when you break your sugar addiction. You will be doubly amazed by how much sugar is added to processed food that you will be able to taste, after you've given up ice cream, cupcakes, cookies, candy and whatever else you've used to satisfy your sugar cravings.

5. **Eliminate bread, pasta and wheat**. This will greatly reduce the fatty calories that you consume when going to restaurants and you're filled with bread before your meal comes. It takes fattening and preservative laden crackers, cupcakes and bagels out of the picture.

6. **Eliminate dairy**. Cheese is the most fattening food we consume next to oil. Milk contains growth hormones which may cause us great harm. Of all the things I may suggest to clients to eliminate, they report they get the greatest benefit from eliminating dairy. Especially those who have suffered from skin diseases, allergies and sluggish digestion.

7. **Drink only water**. Water is the best thing going, but we do not drink enough of it. We are too addicted to drinks with additives, sweeteners and sugar. Gatorade has food colorings, sugar and salt. Soda and energy drinks have added caffeine. Most people drink their coffee with milk and sugar. Then we cap off the evening with a cocktail. Those drinks are normally consumed because of their addictive nature, but dependency on substances to get up and get going, then to calm down after a day's work is done does not buttress your metabolic functioning.

8. **Intermittent fasting**. I know plenty of people who rave about intermittent fasting. Essentially you restrict your meals to a few hours per day. I know people who only eat between noon to 4pm. Some choose a different time slot that may be a six-

hour period, for instance from 3pm to 9pm, which it based on their schedule. Intermittent fasting gives your digestive system a rest and burn and helps to eliminate toxicity.

9. **Go meatless and cheeseless a few days a week**. Many people want to jump into plant-based eating, but they run out of steam in a few days. However, doing it in bite-sized chunks may ease you into positive eating habits. You can institute theme days for your family, such as "meatless Mondays" or "salad Saturdays."

10. **Eliminate alcohol**. Drinking alcohol can be a devasting thing to do metabolically, even if you're not an alcoholic. It wears out your liver, which is the detoxify organ of your body. Also, the activities associated with alcohol can be devasting. I've know many people who have said they can't drink without having a cigarette, which is another potentially devasting habit. I've known others who say they sleep better when they're not drinking. I had one client who I convinced to switch from beer to wine and he started to lose weight immediately. The benefits may be priceless going alcohol free.

11. **Keep lots of fruit in your home**. Buy a huge fruit bowl and fill it with bananas, apples, oranges, mangos, cantaloupe, pears, grapes, etcetera. We covet what we see! If it's in front of you, in your face, you'll consume more of it, especially when it starts to go rancid and you feel like a fool because you didn't partake of it. I usually have much more

than enough, which forces me to eat it. The 1st Aisle recommends at least six pieces of fruit per day, but I normally go beyond ten.

12. **Go processed food free for one day**. This one may be the biggest challenge, but it will be extremely enlightening. Processed food is deadly over the course of your lifetime. Therefore, for one day, don't consume anything bottled, canned, wrapped, hermetically sealed or mass produced in any way. That means you must buy food from the first aisle of the supermarket and prepare it yourself. The only exception would be dried beans and rice, which we'll assume are not processed. Use any cooking method you'd like, but no bottled oil will be used, nor any packaged condiments like salt, sugar or bottled spices (steaming or sautéing with water may be your best options). All ingredients must be straight from the ground, picked from a bush or fallen from a tree. If you take on this challenge you will be surprised at how difficult it may be, but you will be enlightened by how dependent we are on processed food for our existence. However, this may be the biggest step you'll ever take to "optimize" your metabolism.

Appendix F - The Perils of Cooked Food

According to research by Dr. Paul Kouchakoff at the Institute of Clinical Chemistry in Lausanne, Switzerland in the 1930s, cooked food invokes an immune system response when eaten, while raw vegetation does not invoke an immune system response. After eating cooked food, the number of leukocytes (white blood cells) increase, hence the reaction was called digestive leukocytosis. It was also found that eating processed foods (e.g., white flour products, white rice), foods with additives and preservatives, and foods that had been pasteurized (flash heating at high temperatures to kill bacteria) or homogenized (milk where the fat is artificially suspended) also invoked an immune system response. Since the immune system responded similarly to that of a virulent virus, bacteria or pathogen attacking the body, the reaction was renamed "pathological leukocytosis."[88,89, 90]

The topic of "digestive leukocytosis" deserves further investigation because there does not seem to be much follow up research of Dr. Kouchakoff's findings in the 1930s. However, it is undeniable that heating food at high temperatures alters its enzymes and causes abnormal and unnatural processes to occur. We cannot be sure how harmful those abnormal and unnatural process could be, but there is evidence that toxic substances and carcinogens are created and harm the body. Eating as many raw vegetables and fruits as possible could negate the effect of cooked or processed food.

Following are some of the harmful, toxic or carcinogenic compounds formed when food is cooked and processed:

Acrylamides: A caramelization effect that causes carbohydrates to turn brown when heated. Acrylamides are a toxic cancer-causing byproduct of the reaction. Highest risk foods are fried foods like potato chips and French fries; baked snacks with wheat and sugar, like crackers and cookies; and processed grains, like toasted wheat cereals.[91]

Furfural/Furans: Created when sugars are heated. They are toxic and cause skin irritation.

Heterocyclic Amines: Cancerous substances formed when amino acids, sugars, and creatine or creatinine (substances found in muscle) react at high temperatures, such as frying. Heterocyclic amines are usually found in meats like beef, fish and chicken.[92, 93]

Indole and Skatole: Toxic substances found in cooked cheeses. It is produced from tryptophan and found in feces.[94]

Methylglyoxal and Atractylosides: Cancerous toxins produced when heating coffee beans.[95,96]

Nitrosamines: Carcinogenic compounds produced when nitrites and amines combine in acidic places like the human stomach. They are found predominantly in the processes of salting, pickling and curing. High levels of nitrosamines are found in salami, sausages, bologna, ham and bacon. High nitrosamine intake has been linked to gastrointestinal cancers, especially from cured meats, sausages and salted fish.[97,98]

Polycyclic Aromatic Hydrocarbons: Carcinogens formed when fat and juices from meat grilled directly over a heated surface or open fire drip onto the surface or fire, causing flames and smoke. The smoke contains polycyclic aromatic hydrocarbons that then adhere to the surface of the meat.[99]

Hydrogenated Oils/Trans Fats: Man-made fats, also called hydrogenated or partially hydrogenated fats, were created so processed food would not go rancid. They can lead to obesity, heart disease, and other health problems.

ENDNOTES

[1] WHO.int, World Health Organization - Diabetes,
http://www.who.int/mediacentre/factsheets/fs312/en/
[2] USDA-ERS, https://draxe.com/charts-american-diet/
[3] Wikipedia.com, Carl Lewis, https://en.wikipedia.org/wiki/Carl_Lewis
[4] YouTube.com, Carl Lewis: Olympic Medals through the Vegan Diet,
https://youtu.be/bOTETXwflaY?t=2m22s
[5] YouTube.com, Tom Brady Calls Coca-Cola Poison for Kids,
https://youtu.be/h4OXkgZJpjw?t=30s
[6] Health.com, This Drastic Diet Change Helped Venus Williams Fight
Her Autoimmune Condition,
http://www.health.com/nutrition/venus-williams-raw-vegan-diet
[7] BleacherReport.com, THE SECRET (BUT HEALTHY!) DIET POWERING
KYRIE AND THE NBA, http://bleacherreport.com/articles/2744130-the-
secret-but-healthy-diet-powering-kyrie-and-the-nba
[8] YouTube.com, Nike and Kyrie Irving Present: Find Your Groove,
https://www.youtube.com/watch?v=gxC6lkqYyQU
[9] USAToday.com, Veggie might: Titans' D gets boost after going vegan,
https://www.usatoday.com/story/sports/nfl/2017/12/20/veggie-
might-titans-d-gets-boost-after-going-vegetarian/108771904/
[10] American Egg Board, http://www.aeb.org/farmers-and-
marketers/industry-overview
[11] The Washington Post, The U.S. Government is Poised to Withdraw
Longstanding Warnings About Cholesterol,
https://www.washingtonpost.com/news/wonk/wp/2015/02/10/feds-
poised-to-withdraw-longstanding-warnings-about-dietary-
cholesterol/?utm_term=.250709b6c446
[12] Physicians Committee for Responsible Medicine,
http://www.pcrm.org/USDA
[13] Michael Pollan, In Defense of Food, pp. 27-30.
[14] World Health Organization, Food and Agricultural Organization of the
United Nations,
http://www.who.int/nutrition/publications/micronutrients/924159401
2/en/

[15] PubMed.gov, Veganism, Bone Mineral Density, and Body Composition: a study in Buddhist nuns, https://www.ncbi.nlm.nih.gov/pubmed/19350341

[16] National Geographic, What the World Eats, https://www.nationalgeographic.com/what-the-world-eats/

[17] MedicalDaily.com, http://www.medicaldaily.com/75-americans-may-suffer-chronic-dehydration-according-doctors-247393

[18] Time.com, Why Your Bottled Water Contains Four Different Ingredients, http://time.com/3029191/bottled-water-ingredients-nutrition-health/

[19] CaffeineInformer.com, http://www.caffeineinformer.com/harmful-effects-of-caffeine

[20] The Top 15 Caffeine Withdrawal Symptoms, CaffeineInformer.com, http://www.caffeineinformer.com/caffeine-withdrawal-symptoms-top-ten

[21] NationalDairyCouncil.org, Lactose Intolerance Among Different Ethnic Groups, https://www.nationaldairycouncil.org/content/2015/li-among-different-ethnic-groups

[22] ProCon.org, Lactose Intolerance by Ethnicity and Region, http://milk.procon.org/view.resource.php?resourceID=000661

[23] PETA.org, 11 Reasons to Stop Drinking Cow's Milk http://www.peta.org/living/food/reasons-stop-drinking-milk/

[24] MedicalNewsDaily.com, How Much Sugar is in Your Food & Drink, http://www.medicalnewstoday.com/articles/262978.php

[25] American Diabetes Association, http://care.diabetesjournals.org/content/32/4/688

[26] The Truth About Aspartame Side Effects, https://www.healthline.com/health/aspartame-side-effects

[27] Aspartame: The Bitter Truth Behind this Toxic Sweetner, https://www.youtube.com/watch?v=TB6L9S_jc5E

[28] Robert Lustig, MD, Sugar: The Bitter Truth, YouTube, https://youtu.be/dBnniua6-oM

[29]PubMed.com, Water consumption increases weight loss during a hypocaloric diet intervention in middle-aged and older adults, http://www.ncbi.nlm.nih.gov/pubmed/19661958

[30] SugarScience.com, Hidden in Plain Sight, http://www.sugarscience.org/hidden-in-plain-sight/#.WCNs3i0rInR

[31] AuthorityNutrition.com, 10 Similarities Between Sugar, Junk Food and Abusive Drugs, https://authoritynutrition.com/10-similarities-between-junk-foods-and-drugs/

[32] Robert Lustig, MD, YouTube.com, Sugar: The Bitter Truth, https://youtu.be/dBnniua6-oM

[33] National Library of Medicine, Dietary Fructose Consumption Among US Children and Adults, https://www.ncbi.nlm.nih.gov/pmc/articles/PMC2525476/

[34] World Health Day 2016: Action Needed to Halt Rise in Diabetes: http://www.who.int/campaigns/world-health-day/2016/en/

[35] PubMed.com, Obesity and Severe Obesity Forecasts Through 2030: http://www.ncbi.nlm.nih.gov/pubmed/22608371

[36] Health.com, 14 Foods That Make You Look Older, http://www.health.com/health/gallery/0,,20837371,00.html

[37] How the Food Industry Helps Engineer Our Cravings, http://www.npr.org/sections/thesalt/2015/12/16/459981099/how-the-food-industry-helps-engineer-our-cravings

[38] NutritionFacts.org, How Much Fruit is Too Much?, http://nutritionfacts.org/video/how-much-fruit-is-too-much/, 2:30

[39] LiveStrong.com, Eating Fruit Before Meals, http://www.livestrong.com/article/466722-eating-fruit-before-meals/

[40] Mens Health, Best Pre-Workout Foods, http://www.mensfitness.com/nutrition/what-to-eat/best-pre-workout-foods

[41] Time, 50 Healthiest Foods of All Time, http://time.com/3724505/50-healthiest-foods/

[42] The Diet Wars: The Time for Unification Is Now, McDougall Newsletter: August 2012, Volume 11, Issue 8, https://www.drmcdougall.com/misc/2012nl/aug/wars.htm

[43] American Journal of Clinical Nutrition, AJCN.nutrition.org, Nut intake and adiposity: meta-analysis of clinical trials, p. 1346, http://ajcn.nutrition.org/content/97/6/1346.full.pdf

[44] FoodAllergy.org, Facts & Statistics: http://www.foodallergy.org/facts-and-stats

[45] Sydney Local Health District of Australia, http://www.slhd.nsw.gov.au/rpa/allergy/resources/allergy/peanutallergy.pdf

[46] AskDrSears.com, Health Nuts: Ranking Nuts, http://www.askdrsears.com/topics/feeding-eating/family-nutrition/nuts/health-nuts-ranking-nuts

[47] The Starch Solution, John McDougall, MD, Chapter 1, page 3

[48] Eat to Live, Joel Fuhrman, MD, p. 41

[49] The Starch Solution, John McDougall, MD, Chapter 1, Page 15

[50] NutritionFacts.org, The Okinawa Diet: Living to 100, http://nutritionfacts.org/video/the-okinawa-diet-living-to-100/

[51] Federal Food, Drug & Cosmetic Act, http://www.fda.gov/regulatoryinformation/legislation/federalfooddrugandcosmeticactfdcact/

[52] The New York Times, Marian Burros, https://www.nytimes.com/1994/05/05/us/fda-imposing-stricter-rules-on-food-labels.html

[53] The Protein Myth: Why You Need Less Protein Than You Think, http://www.huffingtonpost.com/jessica-jones-ms-rd/protein-diet_b_1882372.html

[54] Nutrition Business Journal, http://www.nutraingredients-usa.com/Markets/NBJ-The-US-supplement-industry-is-37-billion-not-12-billion

[55] "The Supplement Paradox: Negligible Benefits, Robust Consumption", Pieter A. Cohen, MD, JAMA, October 11, 2016, Volume 316, Number 14, p. 1453, https://jamanetwork.com/journals/jama/article-abstract/2565733

[56] New York Times, 4/3/2018, Older Americans are 'Hooked' on Vitamins, https://www.nytimes.com/2018/04/03/well/older-americans-vitamins-dietary-supplements.html

[57] Herbal Supplements Are Often Not What They Seem, http://nyti.ms/1bQ9QbC

[58] DNA Barcoding http://bmcmedicine.biomedcentral.com/articles/10.1186/1741-7015-11-222

[59] Time, http://healthland.time.com/2011/05/25/study-u-s-calcium-guidelines-may-be-too-high/

[60] TheChalkBoardMag.com, http://thechalkboardmag.com/get-dense-why-you-should-be-eating-foods-with-high-andi-scores

[61] NIDDK Digestive Diseases Statistics for the United States https://www.niddk.nih.gov/health-information/health-statistics/Pages/digestive-diseases-statistics-for-the-united-states.aspx

[62] InsiderMonkey.com, 11 Countries with Highest Rates of Osteoporosis in the World, http://www.insidermonkey.com/blog/11-countries-with-the-highest-rates-of-osteoporosis-in-the-world-359037/

[63] Today.com, Calcium Supplement, Dairy, Do Little to Protect Bones, http://www.today.com/health/calcium-supplements-dairy-do-little-protect-bones-t47021

[64] Multivamin Researchers Say "Case is Closed After Studies Find No Benefits", http://www.cbsnews.com/news/multivitamin-researchers-say-case-is-closed-supplements-dont-boost-health/

[65] The Starch Solution, John McDougall, M.D., page 9

[66] Dr. Paul Kouchakoff "The Influence of Food Cooking on the Blood Formula of Man", https://www.conscious-cook.com/dr-paul-kouchakoff-the-influence-of-food-cooking-on-the-blood-formula-of-man/

[67] VeryWellFit.com, Does Cooking Vegetables Increase Their Nutrient Value?, https://www.verywellfit.com/3-vegetables-made-healthier-when-cooked-4057179

[68] Huffington Post, The Protein Myth: Why You Need Less Protein Than You Think, http://www.huffingtonpost.com/jessica-jones-ms-rd/protein-diet_b_1882372.html

[69] The Role of Methionine in Cancer Growth Control, http://www.naturalmedicinejournal.com/journal/2015-12/role-methionine-cancer-growth-and-control

[70] NutritionFacts.org, A Low Methionine Diet May Help Starve Cancer Cells, Sept. 2014, http://nutritionfacts.org/2014/07/08/a-low-methionine-diet-may-help-starve-cancer-cells/

[71] Healthaliciousness.com, Top 10 Foods Highest in Methionine, https://www.healthaliciousness.com/articles/high-methionine-foods.php

[72] Medscape.com, Does Growth Hormone Cause Cancer, http://www.medscape.com/viewarticle/522728_3

[73] HT Health, Why doesn't Europe import U.S. beef?, http://health.heraldtribune.com/2014/07/22/doesnt-europe-import-u-s-beef/

[74] YouTube.com, Are Humans Designed to Eat Meat?, Milton Mills, MD, https://youtu.be/sXj76A9hl-o

[75] Our World Famous McDonald's Fries, https://www.mcdonalds.com/gb/en-gb/product/fries-medium.html

[76] USA McDonald's fries have 14 ingredients. UK McDonald's fries have 4., https://boingboing.net/2015/01/22/usa-mcdonalds-fries-have-14.html

[77] Fox News, McDonald's fries in the US have way more ingredients than UK fries, http://www.foxnews.com/food-drink/2015/01/26/mcdonald-s-fries-in-us-have-way-more-ingredients-than-uk-fries.html

[78] Wall Street Journal, Report Details Dr. Atkin's Health Problems, 2/10/2004, https://www.wsj.com/articles/SB107637899384525268

[79] YouTube.com, Processed Food: An Experiment That Failed, Robert Lustig, MD, https://youtu.be/pvgxNDuQ5DI?t=3m49s

[80] YouTube.com, Processed Food: An Experiment That Failed, Robert Lustig, MD, https://youtu.be/pvgxNDuQ5DI?t=5m39s

[81] Swallow This, Joanna Blythman, p. vii

[82] FoodSafetyNews.com, Processing Aids: What's not on the Label and Why, http://www.foodsafetynews.com/2013/06/processing-aids-whats-not-on-the-label-and-why/#.Wr7cOljwbct

[83] Swallow This, Joanna Blythman, pp. 204-206

[84] BusinessInsider.com, These 10 companies control everything you buy, http://www.businessinsider.com/10-companies-control-the-food-industry-2016-9/#kelloggs-1

[85] Is Sitting the New Smoking?, Forbes.com, https://www.forbes.com/sites/davidsturt/2015/01/13/is-sitting-the-new-smoking/#658b9a234fd4

[86] American Chiropractic Association, Back Pain Facts and Statistics https://www.acatoday.org/Patients/Health-Wellness-Information/Back-Pain-Facts-and-Statistics

[87] National Institute of Health, Fuel Choice During Exercise Is Determined by Intensity and Duration of Activity, https://www.ncbi.nlm.nih.gov/books/NBK22417/

[88] Raw Foods and Enzymes, http://www.healingdaily.com/detoxification-diet/enzymes.htm

[89] NEC Health News, Kouchakoff 2.0, https://wholefoodsmagazine.com/sites/default/files/nechealth_0.pdf

[90] The Influence of Food Cooking on the Blood Formula of Man, First International Congress of Microbiology, Paris, 1930 (edited), https://www.seleneriverpress.com/historical/influence-of-food-cooking-on-the-blood-formula-of-man/

[91] The Worlds Healthiest Foods, What is Acrylamide and How is it Involved with Food and Health?, http://www.whfoods.com/genpage.php?tname=george&dbid=260

[92] PubMed.com, Heterocyclic amines: Mutagens/Carcinogens Produced During Cooking of Meat and Fish, https://www.ncbi.nlm.nih.gov/pubmed/15072585

[93] National Cancer Institute, Chemicals in Meat Cooked at High Temperatures and Cancer Risk,
https://www.cancer.gov/about-cancer/causes-prevention/risk/diet/cooked-meats-fact-sheet#r1

[94] Wikipedia, Skatole, https://en.wikipedia.org/wiki/Skatole

[95] National Institute of Health, Methylglyoxal, the Dark Side of Glycolysis, https://www.ncbi.nlm.nih.gov/pmc/articles/PMC4321437/

[96] National Institute of Health, Methylglyoxal content in drinking coffee as a cytotoxic factor, https://www.ncbi.nlm.nih.gov/pubmed/20722928

[97] EatingforEnergy.com, Nitrates, Nitrites, Nitrosamines,
http://www.eatingforenergy.com/nitrates-nitrites-and-nitrosamine/

[98] Background: Nitrosamines,
http://www.cbc.ca/natureofthings/m_features/background-nitrosamines

[99] National Cancer Institute, Chemicals in Meat Cooked at High Temperatures and Cancer Risk,
https://www.cancer.gov/about-cancer/causes-prevention/risk/diet/cooked-meats-fact-sheet#r1

Made in the USA
Columbia, SC
09 November 2018